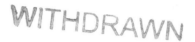

The Exhaustion
Breakthrough

The Exhaustion Breakthrough

Unmask the Hidden
Reasons You're Tired and
Beat Fatigue for Good

HOLLY PHILLIPS, MD

RODALE.

Rodale books may be purchased for business or promotional use or for special sales. For information, please write to:

Special Markets Department, Rodale Inc., 733 Third Avenue, New York, NY 10017

Printed in the United States of America

Rodale Inc. makes every effort to use acid-free ♾, recycled paper ♻.

Illustration by iStock

Book design by Christina Gaugler

Library of Congress Cataloging-in-Publication Data is on file with the publisher.

ISBN 978–1–62336–505–9 hardcover

Distributed to the trade by Macmillan

2 4 6 8 10 9 7 5 3 1   hardcover

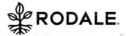

We inspire and enable people to improve their lives and the world around them.
rodalebooks.com

To Olivia and Pascale,
for making every moment magical

Contents

Part I: Fatigue and You:
Assessing Its Impact

Part II: Fighting Fatigue: Lifestyle Factors
That Impact Energy

Part III: Sick and Tired

Part IV: Repairing Your Energy Drains

Acknowledgments

THANK YOU TO MY late father, Myron Phillips, for being who you were, living the way you did, and making me want to be just like you.

I'd like to recognize and express tremendous gratitude to my collaborator, Stacey Colino. Your vision for what this book could be expanded my own, and your resourcefulness, dedication, and countless hours of hard work were awe-inspiring. Thank you for pouring your talent and passion into this project.

I'm truly appreciative of my many mentors and colleagues from Columbia University College of Physicians and Surgeons and Lenox Hill Hospital. Herbert Chase, MD, thank you for your unwavering support when I needed it most and your infectious enthusiasm for this privilege that is the practice of medicine. And thank you, Kay Cynamon, MD, for making sure I never ordered magnesium levels unnecessarily.

Thank you, Bernard Kruger, MD, for opening up your one-of-a-kind practice to me 13 years ago and for making me a part of your incredible family. The way you practice medicine is truly how it should be done, and I'm humbled to be able to learn from you every day. And I'm supremely indebted to my nurse, Agata Was, for helping to solve every mystery diagnosis that comes through our door.

To my fellow journalists, producers, and friends from CBS News, CBS2 News, 48H, and CBS Radio, thank you for allowing me to do what I love for so many years; Susan Schackman, Leigh Ann Winick, Ryan Kadro, Diana Miller, Chris Licht, David Rhodes, Eric Bloom, Mosheh Oinounou, Brian Applegate, Marci Waldman, Chris Zawistowski, Weesie Viera, Susan Zarinsky, Al Briganti, Pam Auerbach, David Friend, Valerie Feder, Kim Godwin, you are all extraordinary. And a special thanks to Sharisse Scineaux and Mary McGeever for teaching me how to turn a package in 10 minutes flat.

To my fantastic team of agents at N.S. Bienstock, thank you for making it happen and keeping it happening: Carole Cooper, Steven Devall, Adam Leibner, Richard Leibner, Samantha Bina, and Julie Clark, I'm so fortunate to have your support. And Paul Fedorko, you took my "eureka" moment, ran with it, and inspired me to run with it, and I'm endlessly grateful.

Of course, no idea becomes reality without opportunity. Thank you to the team at Rodale for believing in this book and making the process seamless and pleasant. Marisa Vigilante, Kristen Kiser, Jennifer Levesque, Aly Mostel, Jess Fromm, you are all appreciated. And many thanks to Lauren Paul, Bethridge Toovell, and the entire group at *Prevention* magazine.

To my NYC friends who are family: I'm so fortunate to have too many to list, but you know who you are. You've made the "Best City in the World" my home.

It's hard to find words to capture my gratitude to my husband, Jose Tavarez. From the moment we met almost 20 years ago, you have been my biggest champion, my most important collaborator, and a superhuman foundation of love and support. Thank you for growing up with me and growing old with me.

And last but far from least, thank you to my patients for inspiring me daily and to my readers for sharing in this journey.

Introduction

DO YOU KNOW A woman who doesn't at least occasionally complain about being tired? I don't. That's true in my busy medical practice, and it's true in my personal life. Most of my conversations with close female friends start like this:

"How are you?"

"Great! Well . . . exhausted, but otherwise great."

"Ugh! Me, too . . ."

We're so accustomed to this shared weariness that we dismiss it like a run-of-the-mill windy day. Sure, the fatigue is a drag on our bodies, minds, and spirits, and yes, it makes life more challenging. But many of us see women's exhaustion as so common, perhaps even unavoidable, that we figure it's not worth talking about. My feeling is, it shouldn't be that way and it doesn't have to be that way, as this book will show you.

Believe me, I'm intimately familiar with this phenomenon, not just as a physician but because I was tired for 20 years straight. During this time, my fatigue was often debilitating. From the moment I woke up, I'd start thinking about how and when I could take a nap. I'd have about 2½ hours of good energy first thing in the morning, then it would wane for the rest of the day, and it had nothing to do with how long I had slept the night before. More often than not, the whole day was a struggle: It was hard for me to get places and often difficult to stay awake. I would pump myself up with caffeine throughout the day; at one point, I was drinking about a pot of coffee daily—that's how I made it through medical school.

As it turns out, I had plenty of good company. Female fatigue has reached epidemic proportions, according to national statistics. In 2010, women across the United States named fatigue among their top five health concerns in WebMD's annual Year in Health survey. A 2013 survey by the Centers for Disease Control and Prevention found that 16 percent of women ages 18 to 44 reported often feeling "very tired" or "exhausted"—responses along the more extreme end of the fatigue spectrum—during the previous 3 months, nearly double the percentage of men who did. The study didn't examine the reasons for the gender disparity, but I suspect men generally feel less fatigue.

Meanwhile, a 2013 survey by the Pew Research Center found that there is (literally!) no job more exhausting than being a mother: While mothers report that it's very meaningful to care for their children, perform housework, enjoy leisure time, and do paid work, they find all of these activities to be more exhausting than men do. Not surprisingly, 45 percent of women reported feeling fatigue due to stress, according to the American Psychological Association's 2012 Stress in America survey. And in 2007, the only year that the National Sleep Foundation's annual Sleep in America poll focused solely on women, 43 percent said that daytime sleepiness interferes with their daily activities.

Women also have more trouble falling asleep and staying asleep than men do, according to the National Sleep Foundation, and they take on more housework and childcare than their male partners, leaving less time for rest. In addition to experiencing exhaustion more often, women consistently report higher levels of fatigue than men do, according to a 2011 study by researchers at Stony Brook University in New York. Making matters worse, some of the most common illnesses in which fatigue is a symptom—such as lupus, thyroid disorders, anemia, celiac disease, irritable bowel syndrome, depression, and rheumatoid arthritis—occur more frequently in women.

The exhaustion epidemic is clearly alive and well among women in the United States, which begs the critical question: *Is it really acceptable that millions of women feel incredibly tired, day in and day out, without the prospect of relief in sight?*

My response to that is *Absolutely not!* This issue should be foremost on the mind of every doctor who treats women. Instead, fatigue is often viewed as an unfortunate fact of a busy woman's life, as unavoidable as elevator music or calls from telemarketers.

When my exhaustion was becoming debilitating while I was a medical student, the doctors I consulted basically said, "Of course you're exhausted—you're in medical school!" Yes, I expected to be as short on sleep and dependent on coffee as any other doctor-in-training, but I knew that my fatigue went well beyond what my peers were experiencing. Simply put, I felt wiped out nearly every hour of every day. Still, I let the prevailing notion that medical students are destined to feel drained discourage me from aggressively seeking treatment. Like so many other women, I bought into the idea that painful exhaustion was the penalty I had to pay for being ambitious and working hard.

Despite the unrelenting fatigue, like most women I simply pushed on with fulfilling my daily responsibilities and pursuing my aspirations. Over the next decade, I went on to become a doctor, a TV medical correspondent, a wife, and a mother. But with the arrival of my second child, I drew a line in the proverbial sand. By this time, I was so sick and tired of being tired that I refused to accept that it was going to be my lifelong reality. I decided then and there to make it my mission to recover and help other women along the way.

Over the course of 15 years, I had been diagnosed with depression, chronic fatigue syndrome, fibromyalgia, recurrent mononucleosis, and sleep apnea. I had consulted dozens of experts, tried myriad treatments from pills to oxygen chambers, and done so much research that my file on fatigue rivaled the thickness of a classified CIA dossier. Looking back, I don't think I had all the criteria for fibromyalgia, but I did have depression, chronic fatigue, and sleep apnea. It's not surprising that many of the symptoms of chronic fatigue syndrome overlap with those of depression. Decreased energy, difficulty concentrating, irritability, feelings of pessimism and helplessness, a lack of interest in things you used to enjoy—these characteristics are true of both conditions. While depression can cause fatigue, in my case I suspect that it worked the other way around—that my exhaustion was taking a toll on my mood. The diagnoses were an important acknowledgment that the fatigue wasn't all in my head, but unfortunately, they didn't add up to a solution right away. Perhaps if I had taken steps to manage my shortage of energy earlier on, I could have avoided the derailing illness of depression altogether.

This frustrating experience stayed with me, and now I'm especially attentive to my own patients who complain of fatigue. The vast majority of those patients who come to my busy Manhattan practice say they feel so run down that the only activity they have a drop of enthusiasm for is sleep. Lying in corpse pose (savasana) at the end of a yoga class is another favorite. *But who has the energy to get to yoga?!* Many of these women begrudgingly drag themselves out of bed in the morning, often with a mild sense of dread about the day ahead. They feel like they're going through the motions in their lives rather than truly living. They keep themselves going with coffee, energy drinks, or other stimulants. Sound familiar?

The truth is that even if your persistent fatigue isn't on the extreme end of the spectrum or a symptom of a major clinical condition, it can still drain the happiness and vitality out of your life. Feeling tired and wiped out is, without question, the most common general health complaint that I hear as a doctor. Yet the women who come to see me rarely make an appointment to address fatigue directly. They are simply too resigned to tiredness as a fact of modern life to view it as a medical issue. (In the Sleep in America poll, 80 percent of the women surveyed said that when they experience sleepiness during the day, they just accept it and keep going.) It's only when I ask a patient specifically about her energy level that she admits how worn out she is. It's not just the kind of run down that comes from a few nights of too-little sleep. These women are truly and perpetually exhausted, drained, or depleted. They feel like their get-up-and-go has gotten up and gone—or they experience frequent waves of fatigue that nearly flatten them. In short, I get the sense that keeping up with their hectic lives leaves them physically, mentally, emotionally, and spiritually spent.

Given everything that you do in a day, of course you're tired. How could you not be? But you don't have to stay that way. Just because you have a demanding job and/or a family, an active social life, and an overflowing plate of other responsibilities and activities doesn't mean you have to accept fatigue as a way of life. You are entitled to feel well and vibrant, which is why it's a mistake to accept fatigue lying down. Instead, you'd be better off viewing it as a wake-up call to take action to reclaim your energy and vitality and kick your exhaustion to the curb. This can be done! It truly is within your power to revitalize yourself and feel better and more energized than ever.

When fatigue is treated properly, we can each have the energy to do what we want and need to do, and we can do it with considerable enthusiasm and verve. Granted, we may never relish cleaning sticky mac and cheese off a high chair or muddy footprints off a carpet—and we may never become US president or fly to the moon. But when we have our vim and vigor restored, we become less focused on merely surviving and more focused on soaring and thriving. Imagine how amazing it would be to wake up in the morning without worrying about how you'll make it through the day—and instead be able to look forward to all that the day has to offer. That would be incredible. And while it may seem like a pipe dream now, it is attainable. During and after medical school, I went through a long, comprehensive process of gradually unmasking the underlying causes of my exhaustion, and I found ways to counteract them one by one. Now I want to show every chronically tired woman that she can do the same.

But before we embark on that journey to greater vitality, it's important to figure out a few things: How did we get to this sorry, sluggish state? Where are the energy drains in our lives, and how can we repair them? And why have we been ignoring them? In other words, why is female exhaustion such a disregarded issue, both in women's own minds and in the medical field?

I believe there are a number of factors that lead women to accept fatigue as their fate. One is the reality that working women with families continue to take on more childcare duties and chores than their partners. Another is the way television and movies portray either a bedraggled and barely-hanging-on working mom as the status quo or the flip side—the superwoman who can manage it all with a smile on her face. Another factor is the false (but damaging) belief among high-achieving women that if we're not pushing our minds and bodies to the limit, we aren't doing enough. These insidious factors can suck the life out of our lives as well as take a toll on our bodies and minds.

Thanks to the widely accepted stereotype of the super-busy, super-tired superwoman, doctors may neglect to ask a worn-out female patient questions about the level and duration of her fatigue or the impact it's having on her, physically and mentally. Even if an exhausted woman were to ask for help—which is rare, in my professional experience—there are a limited number of diagnoses that physicians are trained to pursue routinely. Ironically, the reason for this is that fatigue is associated with a vast range of different diseases, conditions, and syndromes. And if it's not linked to a specific illness, the underlying cause can be a laundry list of combined factors. Without a doubt, diagnosing the cause of persistent fatigue can be daunting—but that's no reason to regard exhaustion as normal or acceptable.

Ideally, all doctors would use a standardized, systematic approach to investigate an individual woman's case of fatigue. And if traditional medicine were unable to neatly categorize and treat a woman's exhausted state, those doctors would be schooled in the many alternative therapies that could provide relief. Since this perfect-world scenario isn't likely to become reality anytime soon, it's currently up to each and every woman to equip herself with the knowledge she needs to walk into a doctor's office, present informed theories about the roots of her exhaustion (based on her personal circumstances), request appropriate testing, and, if necessary, consider forms of complementary or alternative medicine to help her. The best way to do this is to enhance your understanding of fatigue as it applies to your health so you can speak in specific, relevant terms that will compel a doctor to take action and order appropriate tests or more closely assess certain body systems. Yes, this undertaking will add to the burdens of an already overbooked life, but if you give your fatigue the attention it deserves, you'll be rewarded with a higher level of energy that will make every moment more enjoyable and productive.

That's where this book comes in. Throughout these pages, I will guide you through the process of gaining an essential understanding of your exhaustion—and of finding lasting solutions, whether you've been struggling with an energy shortage for weeks, months, years, or decades. Having managed to function at a high level despite suffering major setbacks in my personal life and career due to exhaustion, I know what it's like to keep up with the demands of work and family while feeling as if my gas gauge is on "E." And I'm intimately familiar with the sensation that I'm treading water as vigorously as I can and yet struggling to stay above the surface.

Many women out there will wonder whether they're "tired enough" to merit treatment. Trust me: If you're asking yourself that question, you're tired enough. If you feel tired, you are tired—really!—and your fatigue can quickly trigger a vicious cycle: You may feel like you don't have enough energy to get through the day (or night), so you start to drop things from your schedule or to-do list. Generally, forms of self-care are the first things to go: You stop going to the gym; you stop planning and shopping for healthy meals; you stop doing things just to relax, feel good, or have fun. As a result, you become more run down, your stress levels increase, you have a harder time sleeping, and fatigue gets progressively worse. Inadequate sleep has been linked with nearly every chronic disease—from heart disease and stroke to type 2 diabetes—as well as premature mortality from all causes. It's a dangerous downward spiral.

Because I've lived it and I treat it, I want to help you understand the insidious nature of fatigue, describe the havoc that persistent tiredness wreaks on both our bodies and our minds, and reveal just how drastically it reduces the quality of our lives. When you fully comprehend the devastating effects of exhaustion, not addressing it simply isn't an option. The key to handling it effectively is to gracefully navigate the maze of possible lifestyle and medical-related causes of energy depletion, from illnesses or a poor diet to vitamin deficiencies, sleep disorders, a habit of overexercising, and other factors. In this book, I will lead you through that labyrinth in a way that is manageable and constructive rather than confusing.

Even if there isn't a link between your fatigue and a medical condition, you will discover lifestyle and emotional factors that may be contributing to your exhausted state of existence. Using the fatigue diary and the 7-day fatigue-beating challenge in Chapter 14 will help you with that detective work. You will come away from this book with actionable advice on how to mitigate each fatigue-inducing factor with diet and lifestyle changes and, when appropriate, alternative therapies (such as acupuncture, massage, yoga, and herbal supplements). Like me, a substantial number of readers will find that it takes a combination of traditional and alternative treatments to finally ditch extreme fatigue for good. It's worth the effort to find the magical formula that works for you by developing your personalized energy-boosting plan, as outlined in Chapter 14.

Despite having successfully overcome my own exhaustion, I still don't have the boundless energy of a Broadway actress, and it's unlikely that I ever will. From morning to night, my days are packed, and I seldom get an uninterrupted night's sleep thanks to my wonderful but quite active children. But because I have taken the time to find energy-boosting measures that work for me and are compatible with my hectic life (I'll tell you more about those later), I'm now able to handle the pressure and chaos of my usual responsibilities more effectively. I've even come to enjoy my life more now that I'm fully present for it—or at least every minute that's not spent cleaning up spilled mac and cheese. I want the same for you. I wrote this book with the hope that you can use it as your guide to feel more vibrant than ever.

PART I

Fatigue and You: Assessing Its Impact

CHAPTER ONE

How Tired Are You, Really?

IF YOU'VE PICKED UP this book, you already recognize that you're fairly exhausted. But you may not realize just how tired you really are or recognize the exact ways in which you're exhausted. After all, fatigue can take many forms. One woman feels chronically wiped out with a pervasive tiredness that isn't relieved by getting enough sleep, while another starts the day with plenty of vim and vigor but runs out of energy quickly. Meanwhile, a third woman might have a vague but enduring sense of malaise or listlessness, while another feels physically weak, apathetic, and emotionally vulnerable on a regular basis. The point is, there are many different faces of exhaustion, literally and figuratively speaking.

To address your personal energy crisis and repair the elements that are depleting your vitality, it's important to be sensitive to the specific messages your body is sending. You need to listen closely to what your exhaustion is telling you. Otherwise, how can you possibly expect to reverse your state of depletion and restore your vigor to healthier levels? It's not enough to recognize that your energy balance is out of whack; you need to figure out why it's off kilter. Could it be because you're sick with an underlying medical condition? Could your thought patterns, your stress level, or your general state of mind be dragging and slowing you down? Could lifestyle habits such as your food choices or eating patterns, sleep practices, or exercise routines (or lack thereof) be creating an energy leak that's draining you physically and/or mentally? Or have you created a work or social schedule for yourself that's so demanding that it causes you to run out of fuel without ample opportunities for replenishing your energy reserves?

The first step toward breaking the exhaustion cycle is to identify and understand what is zapping your energy and contributing to your profound sense of fatigue. Then, and only then, can you begin to take steps to revitalize and reclaim your vigor and well-being. So let's start that identification process!

GETTING TO THE BOTTOM OF FATIGUE

First, let's establish a sense of how profound your fatigue is and how it affects you. Read each of the following questions and pick the response that best describes you.

1. Would you say that you become fatigued easily?

    Rarely   Sometimes   Often

2. Is your motivation or desire to do things lower when you feel fatigued?

    Rarely   Sometimes   Often

3. Do you have trouble starting new things?

    Rarely   Sometimes   Often

4. Does your fatigue limit you or cause problems in your life?

    Rarely   Sometimes   Often

5. Does your fatigue interfere with your ability to carry out and fulfill certain responsibilities in your life?

    Rarely   Sometimes   Often

6. Does fatigue affect your work, social, or family life?

    Rarely   Sometimes   Often

7. Has your fatigue affected how you socialize with friends or family or engage in leisure activities?

          Rarely   Sometimes   Often

8. Does your fatigue affect your thinking skills, concentration, communication abilities, or other aspects of mental functioning?

          Rarely   Sometimes   Often

9. Does your fatigue interfere with your ability to function physically?

          Rarely   Sometimes   Often

10. Does exercising give you an enduring sensation of tiredness?

          Rarely   Sometimes   Often

11. Does your fatigue affect your eating or sleeping habits or other aspects of your behavior?

          Rarely   Sometimes   Often

12. Has your fatigue affected how you take care of yourself (with bathing, dressing, and the like)?

          Rarely   Sometimes   Often

13. Has your fatigue affected your sex life?

          Rarely   Sometimes   Often

14. Does fatigue rate among your three most incapacitating symptoms?

          Rarely   Sometimes   Often

15. Do you feel distressed or bothered by your fatigue?

          Rarely   Sometimes   Often

If you answered "often" three or more times, you are in need of an antidote for your exhaustion and could use an infusion of fresh, vibrant energy. Fatigue is taking a serious toll on your life, affecting the way you feel and function, your behavior and attitude. And if it hasn't already, it probably will affect your physical or emotional health in the not-too-distant future.

The same is true if you answered "sometimes" five or more times. This is your wake-up call to take your exhaustion seriously.

If you chose "rarely" for many of your responses, you're not entirely out of the energy-drain zone. There's always room for improvement, and this book will show you how to fix your exhaustion triggers and boost your energy in a sustainable fashion. If, however, you chose "rarely" for every single answer—granted, it's a remote possibility, assuming your responses were honest and accurate—then you might want to pass this book along to a tired friend who could truly benefit from reading it.

Now let's try to pinpoint the patterns and rhythms of your fatigue as well as the lifestyle factors that may be contributing to it. Read the following questions and choose the responses that best describe your exhaustion.

1. At what time(s) of the day is your fatigue *most* pronounced?

   a. Late morning

   b. Midday

   c. Late afternoon

   d. Evening

2. Which of the following statements best describes your sleep-wake patterns?

   a. I often wake up feeling unrefreshed and soon start thinking about if or when I can nap.

   b. I have trouble getting to sleep and/or I wake up with the roosters and have trouble going back to sleep.

   c. I tend to skimp on sleep to get more done during the day and evening hours.

   d. I feel as though I get enough sleep and start the day feeling reasonably rested.

3. Which of the following best describes your eating patterns?

   a. I tend to eat erratically, and my pattern can change from day to day.

   b. I usually skip breakfast but eat lunch and dinner.

c. I eat three square meals a day with lunch or dinner being the biggest meal of the day.

d. I often have multiple small meals throughout the day.

4. How would you describe your food preferences?

a. I'm a junk-food junkie—if it's fried, salty, or sweet, I'll probably love it.

b. I'm a serious carb lover—breads, pastas, and grains are the mainstay of my diet.

c. I'm a meat-and-potatoes kind of gal—I like hearty meals that fill me up.

d. I eat a primarily plant-based diet with moderate portions of lean protein.

5. How stressed out do you feel on a daily basis?

a. I am flirting with stress overload; I feel tense and anxious all the time.

b. I spend much of the day feeling anxious about the challenges and responsibilities I have to deal with.

c. I generally feel calm until something upsetting happens—then my stress level soars.

d. I experience ups and downs in the stress department but feel like I have it under control.

6. How well do you manage your stress?

a. I don't. If anything, it manages me; I often feel like I'm at the mercy of the stresses and strains in my life.

b. So-so. Sometimes I remain calm under pressure, but sometimes I cave into it and feel like a wreck.

c. I try to hold on to my can-do spirit and try to control what I can and let go of what I can't—but sometimes stress gets the upper hand.

d. I carve out at least 10 minutes a day to decompress with meditation, deep breathing exercises, or other relaxation strategies—whether I'm feeling stressed or not.

7. Which of the following best describes your exercise habits?

   a. Erratic at best—often I do little more than move my fork to my mouth.

   b. I spend much of the day sitting at my desk, but I try to go for a daily walk.

   c. I'm an addict—I kill myself at the gym with daily extreme-intensity workouts.

   d. I do moderate-intensity exercise on a regular basis and feel as though it boosts my energy.

8. How do you typically use your spare time?

   a. I try to catch up on all the things I never seem to get done on my to-do lists.

   b. I spend a lot of my so-called downtime trying to recover from exhaustion.

   c. I often worry about work, my finances, my family, or other issues—and find it hard to relax.

   d. I spend time with loved ones and engage in hobbies or other activities I enjoy in order to recharge my batteries.

9. Which of the following is your usual beverage of choice?

   a. I'm a java junkie and often drink coffee or strong tea all day long.

   b. I drink a lot of soda—it's refreshing and sweet, which boosts my mood.

   c. I often count the hours until it's cocktail time and don't focus on fluids until then.

   d. I try to drink water or watered-down juices throughout the day.

10. In a perfect world, which of the following best describes the way you'd like to be able to move through life?

a. I just want to regain the feeling that I can make it through each day without crashing and burning.

b. I want to stop worrying about running out of gas and falling further and further behind on things.

c. I want to feel more in control of my life, my moods, and my energy.

d. I want to feel like a force—strong, capable, unstoppable, really.

Before I tell you how to interpret your responses to these questions, it's worth giving yourself a reality check (or reminder). In the media, the myth of the superwoman or supermom is alive and kicking—but it's a fantasy. It's not real or attainable. It's true that you may know a few women who seem to have mastered the juggling act—they look polished or professional; every aspect of their lives (their homes, their children, their careers, their fitness regimens) seems to be in stellar shape; and they often seem ready, willing, and eager to add more to their already full plate of responsibilities. But think about this: How much do you really know about the inner workings of their lives?

They may have an entourage of help (nannies, housekeepers, personal assistants, chefs, trainers, and so on) at their disposal or the financial resources to continuously make their lives easier. They may have an extensive network of family members and friends who can step in at a moment's notice to help. Or they may work very hard to make it seem this way. Appearances can be deceiving, as we all know, and despite the happy face these perfectly put-together women show to the world, they may be privately grappling with depression, exhaustion, or deeply rooted insecurities. They may feel just as overwhelmed, stressed, or depleted as the rest of us do. So cut yourself some slack before playing the comparison game.

Here's another reality check: Some fatigue is natural and inevitable, especially for women. A modicum of fatigue could be a sign that you're living your life with full engagement and commitment—and you probably wouldn't want it to be any other way. So if you chose mostly d's on this questionnaire, you're actually doing pretty well. If you chose mostly b's or c's, you're in good company among the tired sisterhood who run out of fuel in the afternoon and tend to collapse into bed at the end of the day, feeling worn out, stressed out, and in danger of burning out. If you chose mostly a's, you may already be in that state of utter exhaustion, barely able to drag yourself through the day.

The point here isn't to judge yourself but to get a baseline sense of the level of exhaustion you're dealing with—and what it's trying to tell you. Then you can begin to take steps to recharge your body and mind and reclaim your vitality. The key steps are to track your levels of fatigue in a diary and do a 7-day fatigue-beating challenge (both detailed in Chapter 14). If your eating habits seem to be responsible for at least some of your lethargy, you can upgrade your dietary choices by consuming more fruits, vegetables, whole grains, lean protein, and healthy fats. If sedentary behavior is draining your energy, you'll want to move more and sit less. If insufficient or fragmented sleep is making you tired, it's time to make getting good quality shut-eye a priority by improving your sleep hygiene and consulting a sleep specialist if need be. If excessive stress is pushing you into the exhaustion zone, it's time to get a grip on your stress and find ways to relieve it or manage it better. In the pages that follow, you'll learn more about how these various aspects of your lifestyle can contribute to fatigue and discover how sneaky medical conditions (from anemia to autoimmune diseases, from fibromyalgia to type 2 diabetes) can drain your energy, too.

Armed with this knowledge, you'll be able to develop a customized energy-boosting plan that's likely to work for you, as you'll see in detail in Chapter 14. It doesn't matter how long you've been tired or how severe or mild your fatigue is. What is important is that you identify your current energy drains, repair them, and put an end to exhaustion. It is possible. I did it, and you can, too!

CHAPTER TWO

A Crash Course in Fatigue

NOW THAT YOU KNOW more about the patterns behind your fatigue, it's time to get to the bottom of where it is coming from, what your fatigue is trying to alert you to, and what to do about it. Yes, exhaustion makes you feel awful—that's its job. It's trying to tell you something. But the question is, are you heeding the message? Fatigue, just like pain or fever, is one of your body's primary alarm systems designed to alert you that something is out of whack or just plain wrong. In a healthy person, this is how the fatigue-rest-rejuvenation cycle should work: Let's say you lose sleep and/or vigorously exert yourself physically, mentally, or emotionally, and you are left feeling depleted, weak, weary, or unmotivated. These sensations of feeling sluggish or drained tell you that it's time to rest and recuperate, that this is what your body and mind need to do now. Once you've given yourself a restorative break, exhaustion disappears and your energy levels bounce back to normal.

That's the ideal scenario. But when days, weeks, or months go by and you don't get adequate rest—or it provides little to no relief—fatigue can shift from being uncomfortable to crushing. When that happens, you may start to view every drop of energy you have as a precious resource that should only be spent on the most essential activities. All the "extra" pursuits that make life fun and enjoyable—seeing friends, playing with your kids, reading books, browsing in stores—begin to fall by the wayside, simply because you don't have the energy to do them. When you look in the mirror, you may see a faded-looking version of yourself.

The trouble is, fatigue is nearly impossible to sum up in a single sentence, and there is currently no official medical definition for it (the same is true of exhaustion, a term that I am using interchangeably with fatigue). Part of what makes fatigue so complex is that while it is often a symptom that can be caused by a wide range of medical conditions and lifestyle factors, it can also be a medical condition in its own right, as in the case of unexplained fatigue and chronic fatigue syndrome, a complex, debilitating disorder that's marked by overwhelming fatigue and symptoms like muscle pain, impaired memory, and insomnia. The symptoms don't improve with bed rest and tend to worsen after physical or mental exertion. Many narrow medical definitions of fatigue frame it in terms of reduced muscle performance after intense exercise or impaired cognitive ability after extended periods of concentration.

But neither of those fully captures the essence of true fatigue, in my way of thinking. For the purposes of this book, the following definitions, from an article in *Arthritis Care & Research,* may hold the most accurate and relevant distinction between tiredness and fatigue: Tiredness is considered "a universal sensation" and a "natural response" that is expected to occur "at certain times of the day or after certain types of activity or exertion" or due to busy schedules or emotional stress. Fatigue, by contrast, is "an uncommon, abnormal, or extreme whole bodily tiredness which is not related to activity or exertion"; it is more severe than the usual tiredness, and it is often the first symptom of a disease or illness. This distinction will ring true to anyone with fatigue who consistently feels as if everything she does takes more effort than it should, both mentally and physically.

FATIGUE: A SCIENTIFIC PUZZLE

Believe it or not, the research file on fatigue is surprisingly slim. The first medical journal to focus exclusively on fatigue was launched in June 2013 (yes, that recently!). After doing a thorough review of the literature that was published on the subject between 2002 and 2011, the journal's founder, Fred Friedberg, PhD, professor of psychiatry and behavioral science at New York's Stony Brook University, concluded that there are no central theories guiding the study of fatigue, and that too few efforts are being made to discover how it works across diseases, syndromes, and conditions. Indeed, studies on fatigue are so lacking in structure and authority that Dr. Friedberg felt they couldn't yet be described as a field of discipline. Fortunately, the future is brightening: Interest in exhaustion is on an upswing, perhaps due in part to the medical community's increased acceptance of chronic fatigue syndrome, and perhaps because general fatigue is such a prevalent symptom in our society. Either way, some revealing and helpful research is beginning to emerge.

To start unraveling the mysteries of fatigue, researchers are attempting to pinpoint its biology—a huge undertaking given the possibility that each of its psychological, physiological, behavioral, and social components may have its own underlying mechanism. But if scientists are successful in identifying specific organic processes that are responsible for creating or exacerbating fatigue, they may also be able to find ways to interrupt those processes and lessen (or, dare we hope, eliminate) their effects. A handful of trailblazing scientists are already making headway in this pursuit. A few of the promising suspected contributors that are under investigation: Corticotropin-releasing hormone is a hormone that can be knocked out of whack in either direction by chronic stress, and these changes can trigger depression or fatigue. Alterations in mood-regulating hormones such as serotonin and tryptophan can also induce fatigue. Molecules called cytokines that are released during inflammation have been linked with exhaustion. Several neurotransmitters (brain chemicals that transmit signals to nerve cells and other cells in the body), including an especially interesting one called substance P, are found in increased levels in fibromyalgia patients (a disease in which severe fatigue is a primary characteristic, along with widespread pain, sleep disturbances, and cognitive problems).

Additional research is pointing a finger at abnormalities found in the hypothalamic-pituitary-adrenal axis (a major part of the endocrine system that regulates reactions to stress and several body processes, including digestion, immunity, mood and emotions, and sexuality, as well as energy storage and expenditure) and dysfunction of the basal ganglia (deep brain structures that help start and control movement). Many of these research efforts seem promising and are likely to shed more light on understanding fatigue-related conditions, which will hopefully lead to better treatments down the road.

The task of studying patients' experiences with fatigue also can be challenging to scientists because, unlike investigations involving specific substances or systems in the body, the subjectivity of patient reports makes these studies difficult to replicate and therefore validate. Simply put, the sensation of fatigue is a purely personal experience and impossible to measure with a lab test or on a standardized scientific scale. This makes it tricky to compare large numbers of patients and draw conclusions, as is done in classic research trials and clinical studies. Nonetheless, various approaches to studying fatigue have led to some intriguing findings. One is that even individuals with different diseases tend to experience the same physical, cognitive, and social symptoms of fatigue such as cutting back on physical activities, having trouble concentrating, and losing touch with social contacts.

For example, I recently treated a 44-year-old woman who was complaining of fatigue. She happens to be a doctor with a young child, and she was so perpetually exhausted that she cut off social contact with friends and family and now does "nothing that's not mandatory." She was eventually found to have hypothyroidism, a condition in which the body doesn't have enough thyroid hormone. In addition to fatigue, the condition causes weakness, weight gain, cold intolerance, constipation, muscle cramps, and other unpleasant symptoms. Another patient—a 34-year-old mother of three who is an editor at a fashion magazine—told me she would chew on coffee grounds in her office before having to lead a meeting. Her energy was so depleted that she would wake up every morning afraid of what she wouldn't be able to accomplish that day and dreading how painful it would be to try to push through the fatigue. She was eventually diagnosed with chronic fatigue syndrome. Here were two women, 10 years apart in age, with different professions and life circumstances—both suffering with similar symptoms of exhaustion, albeit brought on by different medical conditions.

The Ripple Effect of Fatigue

When exhaustion strikes, it can knock you off your equilibrium or take you down for the count with a barrage of various symptoms that may not even seem related to fatigue. While you might connect muscle weakness with an overall sense of tiredness, you may not make the connection to shortness of breath, sluggish digestion, random aches and pains, frequent sinus or respiratory infections, or migraine headaches. In addition, your brain may get foggy, making it harder to solve problems, make decisions, process what you are reading or hearing, or even remember the word for an object that you encounter countless times every day.

You're more likely to feel emotional distress, depression, and anxiety when faced with minor challenges. In spite of being worn out, you may have trouble falling or staying asleep. Interest in sex might plummet along with your energy levels, and exercise can either help you feel better or make you feel worse.

Extreme fatigue was the common denominator in both conditions, and in both cases it was treated successfully with the right interventions for each diagnosis.

Even within the same disease, the level of fatigue can be quite variable from one person to another. In fact, how exhausted a patient feels may have no direct correlation with the physical severity of his or her illness. In other words, one woman with mild anemia might feel completely wiped out, while another woman with the same level of anemia might feel fine. All of these findings emphasize the multifaceted and often confounding nature of fatigue—a reality that makes finding a cure all the more challenging.

THE ORIGINS OF FATIGUE

It may help to think of your energy reserve as a bank account—one that you make deposits into (with good-quality sleep, a nutritious diet, exercise, proper breathing, healthy relationships, satisfying activities, and so on) and one you make withdrawals from (by being overscheduled, experiencing stress overload, sleeping inconsistently, eating irregular meals, exercising excessively, or, conversely, engaging in too many sedentary activities and the like). When the balance of energy goes too low—when you're making more withdrawals than deposits, in other words—exhaustion sets in and you also may experience fatigue-related symptoms such as depression, digestive distress, lowered resistance to infection, headaches and other pain flare-ups, and other signs of depletion. This is your body's way of telling you that you need to make some substantial deposits in the energy bank—that it's time to rest and recharge, rejuvenate, and replenish your energy reserves in order to stay healthy and feel and function at an optimal level.

Even if you have healthy lifestyle habits, your body naturally goes through energy and fatigue cycles thanks to its internal biological clock. This master timekeeper, located in a region called the suprachiasmatic nuclei

(SCN) in the hypothalamus of the brain, regulates your circadian rhythms—physical, mental, and behavioral changes that roughly follow a 24-hour cycle. Circadian rhythms are influenced by exposure to light and darkness in the environment, which causes cells in the SCN to send signals to other parts of the brain that control the release of hormones (such as cortisol, which energizes you, and melatonin, which makes you sleepy), heart rate, body temperature, and other bodily functions. These natural biological rhythms explain why you are probably more alert in the midmorning and experience an energy dip (perhaps even a bout of sleepiness) between 1:00 and 3:00 in the afternoon (siesta time in some parts of the world). These daily fluctuations also affect your physical strength and endurance, your pain sensitivity, the keenness of your senses, and more. If you're a morning person (a lark) or a night person (an owl), these highs and lows may be slightly earlier or later in the day.

In women, monthly hormonal shifts (thanks to the menstrual cycle and perimenopause, for example) can increase our susceptibility to fatigue as well as our moods. Specifically, fluctuations in estrogen and progesterone can have a trickle-up or trickle-down effect on various body systems—not just our reproductive systems but our cardiovascular, digestive, immune, and nervous systems as well. In addition, they influence the activity of mood- and energy-regulating brain chemicals (like serotonin). As a result, these hormonal shifts may affect our energy levels, our sense of vitality, the quality and quantity of our sleep, and how we feel and function in myriad ways. If you suffer from PMS, you are undoubtedly familiar with these changes. The point is, as women, we have several sets of biological rhythms—including our daily circadian rhythms and our monthly hormonal cycles—that are acting simultaneously; one set can mitigate the effects of the other, or one set can compound the other's effects. It's like an intricate ballet inside your body.

On top of these physiological factors, our lifestyles can influence how energized or exhausted we feel. The issue of not getting enough sleep is the most obvious culprit, but more subtle habits and behaviors affect the energy equation as well. In women, some of the most common energy-depleting factors are an excess of stress, overexercising or being too sedentary, poor nutrition, shallow breathing, poor posture, being a workaholic, procrastinating, and engaging in bad emotional habits such as ruminating about your problems, getting angry easily (or repressing anger), or sending yourself on frequent guilt trips. Individually, each of these can create a considerable energy drain; collectively, they add up to a substantial loss of vitality, one that's akin to a gaping hole in a tire rather than a pinhole-size leak that lets the air out. What's more, lifestyle issues such as work stress or sleep disturbances (courtesy of a snoring husband or a restless cat at your feet) often lead to fatigue; in addition, psychiatric conditions such as depression and anxiety can send you down a path to exhaustion.

Meanwhile, various medical conditions—ranging from anemia to autoimmune diseases to diabetes to lung, kidney, or liver disorders—also trigger fatigue. While these conditions usually result in a constellation of symptoms, fatigue is often one of the first and most prominent.

The truth is, exhaustion is associated with hundreds of physical illnesses and conditions, ranging from life-threatening cardiovascular disease to a simple vitamin deficiency. Fatigue is a common side effect of antihistamines, statins, and other medications. It can be the result of medical treatments such as chemotherapy. Food allergies like gluten intolerance and environmental factors such as carbon monoxide poisoning are fatigue triggers, too. And sometimes, crippling and chronic tiredness sets in for no clear reason and is categorized as "unexplained" or, based on other symptoms that are present, diagnosed as chronic fatigue syndrome or fibromyalgia. With so many possible causes of fatigue, unmasking the specific source of yours may seem daunting. That's just what this book is for: It will give you a clear, step-by-step approach to uncovering the root of your fatigue, and then guide you toward its cure.

TOO TIRED TO FIGHT FATIGUE?

When you're already exhausted, you may feel too tired to investigate, much less try to remedy, your fatigue. To be honest, it took me several years to muster the energy to look for more energy. Just as I did, you might wonder: With so many variables to consider, how can someone who's searching for the source of her fatigue figure out where to start? It can be an exhausting undertaking, which is why I included a series of questionnaires in the previous chapter. These will help you determine the duration and severity of your exhaustion, pinpoint the times of day and situations when it tends to wax and wane, identify your own fatigue-related symptoms, and assess the degree to which fatigue negatively impacts your life. These are all valuable pieces of information that can provide a doctor with clues as to what might be at the root of your exhaustion. They will also help you embark on your own road to greater vitality in the meantime.

When a doctor sees a patient who is complaining of fatigue, the first step is to explore the possibility of an underlying medical condition or contributing lifestyle factor. With thorough examination and testing, some causes will reveal themselves quickly. In women, exhaustion is frequently the result of viral syndromes (such as Epstein-Barr), medications that cause fatigue (such as beta-blockers, diuretics, antihistamines, asthma drugs, and lots of others), thyroid disease, iron deficiency or anemia, depression, sleep disorders, or a multitude of stressors from a toxic work environment to financial hardship to caring for sick or aging family members. All of these possibilities should be discussed during your initial visit, and I'll go into more detail about all of this in later chapters.

If, after a complete workup, a diagnosis remains elusive, your fatigue will be declared "unexplained." If that happens, you'll be in good company. An often cited study from 1990 found that blood tests lead to a diagnosis in just 5 percent of patients complaining of fatigue lasting at least 1 month, a result that makes some doctors hesitant to perform comprehensive lab (or blood) tests. But at the very least, these tests are an extremely useful part of the process of elimination: Even if a cause for a woman's fatigue isn't revealed immediately on a blood test, some potentially serious medical conditions can be ruled out and the doctor and patient can look toward other possible culprits.

The one-third of patients who end up with "unexplained" fatigue still do find significant relief for their exhaustion. A recent review of medical research concluded that the most effective course of treatment for fatigue that has no clear medical causes is a carefully tailored one that meets the patient's unique needs and includes psychological and pharmacological elements as well as an exercise program. One version of this treatment might combine cognitive behavioral therapy with the stimulant modafinil (used to treat excessive daytime sleepiness or narcolepsy) and a daily 30-minute walk. Granted, exercise may seem like a counterintuitive treatment when you're trying to eliminate exhaustion—and it's probably the last thing a tired person feels like doing!—but inadequate physical activity has been shown to worsen the symptoms of fatigue.

In addition to conventional medicine, alternative therapies can help. These range from more commonplace therapies like massage and acupuncture to more unusual approaches like spending time in an oxygen chamber (Michael Jackson may have been onto something with this). Several alternative techniques—including acupuncture, mindfulness-based stress reduction, and yoga—are backed by significant research. Others, such as aromatherapy and hydrotherapy, are so low risk and affordable that you may decide they're worth exploring despite a lack of scientific backing. There's no harm in trying them, and they very well might help. Dietary and herbal supplements are a stickier subject: Even if there is compelling evidence in their favor, lack of regulation by the FDA makes issues related to purity/contamination and adverse reactions serious concerns. Before using any alternative treatment, you should discuss the risks and benefits in detail with your doctor.

It's crucial to take the time to find a doctor who will be invested in your health and well-being, one with whom you feel comfortable sharing information and asking countless questions. It's a mistake to play doctor on yourself. Yes, the chapters that follow in this book will help you gain essential insight into your fatigue, including the possible causes of and treatments for it. But no amount of information can take the place of a physician who is willing and eager to do whatever it takes to bring you back to a state of complete health. The best way to conquer fatigue and feel more vibrant than ever involves working closely with your doctor to identify your personal energy drains—and repair them.

PART II

Fighting Fatigue: Lifestyle Factors That Impact Energy

CHAPTER THREE

Night Moves: Improving Sleep Habits

ONE OF MY PATIENTS, Andrea, is a newly married, high-powered Wall Street executive in her early forties. She sleeps 4 hours a night and says she wakes up "naturally," which she interprets as a sign that she just doesn't require much sleep. Yet Andrea complains about never being able to relax, having "constant worry and anxiety," and being "brutally cranky" with her spouse over mundane household matters (like his leaving the toilet seat up). She didn't see these behavior changes and symptoms as signs of exhaustion—but they are. I told her this and suggested she take steps to improve the length and quality of her sleep. At first, she was reluctant to spend more time sleeping because she was so focused on getting things done. But she gradually decided to try to improve the quantity and quality of her sleep for the sake of her mood and her marriage. With the help of meditation, cognitive behavioral therapy (to cope with anxiety), and aromatherapy, within a matter of weeks Andrea noticed an improvement in her state of mind.

We live in a culture where many people, like Andrea, operate according to the principle that "if you snooze, you lose." I see this frequently among patients in my practice, coworkers in the TV world, and my friends. Some high-achieving people who manage to get by on very little shut-eye even view it as a point of pride, or a badge of honor, that *they* can cram more into their days than the rest of us.

Getting insufficient sleep has practically become part of our modern lifestyle—and it has wide-ranging effects on both a personal and a societal level. In the most recent Behavioral Risk Factor Surveillance System survey by the Centers for Disease Control and Prevention (CDC), which included 74,751 adult respondents, 38 percent reported unintentionally falling asleep during the day at least once in the preceding month, and 5 percent reported nodding off or falling asleep while driving at least once in the preceding month. The US Department of Transportation estimates that drowsy driving is responsible for 1,550 fatalities and 40,000 nonfatal injuries each year in the United States—a serious threat to public health!

On a more personal health note, what many of these chronic undersleepers may not realize is that eventually, if they don't snooze long enough or well enough on a regular basis, they will pay a price with their health, well-being, and/or functionality. That's because sleep isn't an inactive state as experts used to believe.

On the contrary, sleep is a highly restorative process that allows you to recover from the previous day and prepare for the next one; think of sleep as a forced time-out for the body and mind. While you're asleep, hormones, including human growth hormone, are released to regulate metabolism, organ function, appetite, and the growth, maintenance, and repair of muscles, tissues, and bones throughout the body. While you're sleeping, your immune system is fortified. Your heart and vascular system get a much-needed rest during non-REM sleep. Then your heart rate, breathing rate, and blood pressure can rise and fall during REM (rapid eye movement) sleep, a phenomenon that seems to improve cardiovascular health. A good night's sleep assists with learning because long-term memories are consolidated and embedded while you slumber. Meanwhile, as you snooze, your skin renews itself, shedding old cells and replacing them with new ones, and important neurotransmitters (brain chemicals) that affect everything from your mood to your senses of hunger and fullness after eating are released. And sleep allows us to conserve energy—as evidenced by the fact that both body temperature and calorie-burning decrease during sleep—which leaves us feeling reinvigorated the next day.

On a very basic level, most of us know that after a good night's sleep we feel more alert and focused, more energetic, more upbeat and capable, and better able to function. But we may not realize the extent to which chronic sleep loss or sleep problems can compromise our physical health and emotional well-being. Ongoing sleep loss has been linked with an increased risk of high blood pressure, heart disease, type 2 diabetes, kidney disease, and stroke. It increases your chances of gaining weight because sufficient sleep helps maintain a healthy balance of the hormones (namely, ghrelin and leptin) that regulate appetite and feelings of fullness; when you don't get enough sleep, levels of these hormones get out of whack, which is why you may feel hungrier (and crave starchy carbohydrates, in particular). Sleep also affects how your body responds to insulin, which in turn controls your blood sugar; hence, chronic sleep loss can lead to elevated blood sugar levels, increasing your risk for diabetes.

On an emotional level, sleep deprivation increases your risk of developing depression or anxiety or being particularly reactive to stress. In fact, in a 2013 study involving 3,374 adults, researchers from the University of Saskatchewan in Canada found that those who cut back on sleep over a 7-year period experienced increased mood instability over time; this was especially noteworthy because people's moods generally become more stable as they get older. Another risk: If you're sleep deprived, you may have difficulty solving problems, making decisions, or controlling your emotions and behavior.

CHALLENGES TO WOMEN'S SLEEP

A variety of factors uniquely affect women's sleep—hormonal fluctuations and the stress of juggling work and family responsibilities are probably at the top of the list. Hormonal changes during the premenstrual phase of our cycles, as well as during pregnancy and the menopausal transition, may affect our sleep patterns, reactions to stress, and our moods. During the premenstrual phase, many women have trouble falling asleep, staying asleep, or waking up when they're supposed to. In fact, insomnia—and the agitation that often comes with it—is one of the most common symptoms of PMS.

Pregnancy can lead to sleep disturbances, especially during the first trimester (when high levels of progesterone tend to make a woman sleepy during the day while disrupting her sleep at night) and the third trimester (when general physical discomfort, heartburn, leg cramps, and lower-back pain can kick in as a woman's belly gets bigger).

Sleep disturbances become more common during the menopausal transition: As estrogen levels drop, night sweats (hot flashes that occur at night) often awaken women, and sleep may be lighter than it was previously. While hormone replacement therapy is rarely used for menopausal symptoms these days, a combination of relaxation therapies, herbal remedies, and exercise may help with hormonal sleep disturbances. Breathing difficulties and snoring also may become more common at this stage of life.

For women of any age, the stress of balancing work and family obligations may contribute to sleep disturbances—and the exhausted or frazzled state of mind that results from them. Many women skimp on sleep in order to get more done. Sure, they're tired, but they try to ignore their fatigue or push through it. Eventually, it catches up with them and they feel wiped out. I see this frequently with my patients. Recently, I treated a married woman who is in her late thirties, has three school-age kids, and is starting her own clothing design business. She asked me for medication to treat attention deficit disorder because she "just can't focus." The real problem, as I saw it, was that she slept only 4 to 5 hours a night, often in fragments. When I suggested that her inability to focus may stem from fatigue and that she try to get more sleep, she explained that she wants to be able to function on minimal sleep because so many of her friends do it. It's almost as if she's competitive about the challenge, but this isn't the kind of race you want to sign up for.

GAINING SNOOZE CONTROL

The first step for anyone who feels like she's running on empty should be to improve her sleep hygiene—even if the cause of her exhaustion is due to another factor like hormonal changes. That means making sleep a priority by allocating enough time to regularly get the optimal amount of shut-eye that you need to feel and function at your best. When life is busy and you feel overextended, overwhelmed, and overly stressed, it's natural to want to stay up later or get up earlier than usual to try to accomplish more during your waking hours. While that strategy may help you chip away at your to-do list in the short run, it will take a toll on your energy, health, and well-being over time—so resist the urge to skimp on sleep. You'd be better off saying no to nonurgent requests, delegating tasks, or setting appropriate limits with others so you can get the rest you need. While sleep needs vary, most adults require 7 to 9 hours per night.

The best way to determine how much sleep *you* need is to do a little experiment: First, try to catch up on sleep for several nights on a weeklong vacation during which you can turn in when you're tired and wake up without an alarm clock. Once your sleep debt has been replenished, keep track of the amount of sleep you need each night after that (nights 5 through 7, for example) to feel alert and energized for the bulk of the next day. You can use this number as a gauge of how much sleep you really require on a regular basis.

When you return home from vacation, make it a priority to carve out enough time for that restorative shut-eye nightly. To reach that optimal quota, adjust your sleep schedule gradually in 15-minute (or no more than 30-minute) increments over a few days: You might shift your bedtime 15 to 30 minutes earlier on a Monday, spend 3 or 4 nights adjusting to the change, then make another shift on Thursday or Friday, and so on—until you're getting the amount of shut-eye that's optimal for you.

To improve the quality and quantity of your sleep every night, try the following strategies.

+ **Stick with a consistent sleep schedule.** That means going to bed and waking up at the same time every day. On weekends, you can vary your sleep schedule slightly, but try to keep the difference to 1 hour or less. Otherwise, staying up late and sleeping in on weekends can disrupt your body's circadian (sleep-wake) rhythms, giving you the equivalent of jet lag without even leaving home.

+ **Make your bedroom a sleep-inducing sanctuary.** It should be dark, quiet, and cool, with a comfortable, supportive mattress and pillows on your bed. To keep out unwanted light, consider installing blackout shades or heavy curtains. Block outside noise by installing double- or triple-pane windows, wearing earplugs, or using a "white noise" machine or one that generates soothing sounds that supposedly entrain your brain waves to reach delta (stage 3 or 4) sleep. Keep the bedroom cool (many people prefer a temperature between 60 and 72 degrees) and well ventilated, using a fan if need be.

+ **Expose yourself to natural light.** Spending time outside, even on a cloudy day, will help keep your body's internal clock ticking properly and help you maintain a healthy sleep-wake cycle. It's best if you can expose yourself to natural light for at least 20 minutes first thing in the morning—by throwing open the curtains, sitting in a sunny window, or using a dawn simulator light or alarm clock.

+ **Steer clear of heavy meals in the evening.** Having a large, spicy, rich, or fatty meal too close to bedtime can interfere with sleep and give you a whopping case of indigestion that keeps you up when you'd like to be snoozing. It's best to finish dinner a few hours before bedtime; if you get hungry later in the evening, have a light snack with sleep-inducing foods that contain tryptophan (an amino acid the brain uses to make calming serotonin). Good choices include whole grain crackers and cheese, cereal and a glass of milk, or a handful of almonds and a banana. Having a cup of caffeine-free chamomile tea can also put you in the mood to snooze.

♦ **Avoid sneaky stimulants that interfere with sleep.** As you probably know, caffeine can keep you up at night, which is why it's best to avoid having coffee, tea, chocolate, and soda for 4 to 6 hours before bedtime. Similarly, the nicotine and other chemicals in cigarettes can rev you up, so avoid these in the evenings if you do smoke. While having a glass of wine or a cocktail (or two or three) can certainly make you sleepy, after a few hours of sleep, alcohol acts as a stimulant, leaving you susceptible to micro- (or full) arousals or awakenings and poorer overall quality sleep as the night goes on. This is another reason why it's best to limit alcohol consumption to no more than one or two drinks per day and to avoid it close to bedtime.

One of my patients is a 28-year-old fashion executive who sleeps 7 to 8 hours a night, which should be enough for many people her age, but she always feels exhausted. When we began discussing her lifestyle in detail, I discovered that she goes out to dinner and then meets friends at bars or lounges almost every night; she typically has three or four cocktails each night, but she says they don't make her feel intoxicated because she consumes them slowly over the course of several hours. She loves her lifestyle—and describes it as very *Sex and the City*—so it took some persuasion to convince her to try going 2 weeks without alcohol. My suspicion was that the alcohol was disturbing her sleep as her body metabolized it, resulting in less restorative sleep and more microarousals, causing her to awaken in a state of mild dehydration in the morning. For 2 weeks, she became a teetotaler and reported that she slept more soundly than ever and her energy level doubled. Because she didn't want to give up her lifestyle, she decided to cut back on the frequency, rather than the quantity, of her drinking so she could have several nights of "good sleep" per week—a change that improved her energy level overall.

♦ **Exercise during the day.** Playing sports or working out can set you up for a good night's sleep—but the timing matters for some people. It's best to finish vigorous workouts by late afternoon to give your body temperature, heart rate, and other functions enough time to drop, postexercise, to set the stage for sound slumber. In fact, the 2013 National Sleep Foundation's Sleep in America poll, which included 1,000 adults between the ages of 23 and 60, found that people who exercise vigorously in the morning have the best sleep patterns, including better-quality sleep and a lower likelihood of awakening feeling unrefreshed. It's fine to do relaxing exercises like yoga or simple stretching in the evening.

♦ **Banish technology from your bedroom.** Don't bring your laptop, your smartphone, or other high-tech gadgets to bed with you. The light alone from these devices can reset your body's internal clock; plus, using these devices tends to be stimulating, which isn't what you want before you turn in for the night. So unplug, shut it down, or turn it off. (Your bed partner will thank you.)

♦ **Give yourself a chill-out period before bed.** Avoid strenuous or stimulating activities or emotionally upsetting conversations in the hours before climbing into bed. Physically and psychologically stressful activities trigger the release of cortisol in your body, which increases alertness and arousal. Instead, establish a relaxing bedtime routine—taking a warm bath, doing some gentle stretches, listening to calming music, and the like—before going to bed. Also, be sure to dim the lights: Spending time in bright artificial light—from a TV or computer screen, for instance— tells your brain to stay alert rather than get sleepy.

♦ **Be smart about napping.** The truth is, napping can be a double-edged sword. Yes, a nap during the day may serve as a welcome pick-me-up, boosting energy, alertness, and productivity. But if you struggle with falling asleep or staying asleep at night, daytime napping will likely disturb

The Quest for Rest

Rest isn't a substitute for sleep—but the converse is true as well. Your body needs plenty of sleep *and* periods of rest on a daily basis. Think of rest as another way to recharge your batteries and reboot your body's energy systems. In his book *The Power of Rest: Why Sleep Alone Is Not Enough,* Matthew Edlund, MD, a sleep specialist, makes a case for how and why we all need more active forms of rest, too, in order to stave off feelings of depletion and depression and help our hearts, minds, and central nervous systems work optimally. Here are four energy-boosting ways to rest, other than sleeping:

- ◆ **PHYSICAL REST:** Active forms of rest are conscious and goal oriented. They rely on basic bodily processes to calm and rejuvenate your body and mind—through deep breathing, muscle relaxation exercises, or certain yoga poses, for example.

- ◆ **MENTAL REST:** Calming and focusing your mind in ways that are relaxing and rejuvenating enhances your mood, creativity, and energy level. Good ways to do this: visualization exercises, self-hypnosis, and meditation.

- ◆ **SOCIAL REST:** Human beings are social creatures, so spending time with people who are supportive, interesting, and fun loving, and with whom you have a meaningful connection, is stress relieving, health promoting, inspiring, and energizing.

- ◆ **SPIRITUAL REST:** Whether you reinvigorate your soul with prayer, contemplative thought, or time spent in nature, this type of rest helps you gain valuable perspective and a sense of meaning in your life—and it can give you an infusion of vitality.

your nighttime sleep patterns even more. If you do decide to nap, it's best to take it by midafternoon and limit it to no more than 30 minutes.

- **Kick your pets out of bed.** Research suggests that the number of people who let their pets sleep in their beds yet find their animals disturb their sleep is on the rise. As much as you love your dog or cat, it's not worth sacrificing precious sleep to be near them. Train your pet to sleep on his or her own bed on the floor—or outside your room. Similarly, if your partner tosses and turns, kicks, snores, or otherwise disturbs your sleep on a regular basis, you may want to consider having separate beds. You can still have a strong, loving relationship without sleeping together; in fact, your relationship may even improve if you're both well rested.

- **Get out of bed if you can't sleep.** Don't lie awake counting sheep or worries or staring at the clock; get up, go to another room, and read or do something relaxing or monotonous until the mood to snooze returns. Otherwise, you could come to associate your bed with *not sleeping*— exactly what you don't want to happen!

THE MYSTERIES OF SLEEP DISORDERS

If you can't improve your sleep patterns on your own or if you find that you continuously wake up feeling far from refreshed despite logging enough hours in bed, it may be time to consult a sleep specialist. The reality is, sleep disorders—such as insomnia, sleep apnea, and restless legs syndrome—are more common than many people think. Trust me, because I know: During the worst phase of my own exhaustion, a sleep study revealed that I have mild obstructive sleep apnea, even though I don't have the body type that's typical of this disorder. Simply put, my brain and body weren't getting enough air during the night, which is part of the reason I constantly felt wiped out.

Approximately 70 million people in the United States suffer from chronic sleep problems, according to the CDC, and women are twice as likely as men to have trouble falling asleep or staying asleep. The most common sleep disorders are insomnia (difficulty falling or staying asleep), sleep apnea (breathing interruptions during sleep), and restless legs syndrome (a tingling or creepy-crawly sensation in the legs). There are others that aren't as common—such as circadian rhythm sleep disorder, shift work sleep disorder, REM sleep behavior disorder, narcolepsy, teeth grinding, and others—but I'm going to address only the most prevalent ones here.

Insomnia: When we think of insomnia, many people envision a night spent tossing and turning. But insomnia takes many forms: Some people have trouble falling asleep; others have trouble staying asleep and awaken one or more times during the night and then struggle to get back to sleep; still others wake up too early in the morning, before they've had enough sleep, and can't go back to sleep. Insomnia can be acute (or transient) or it can be chronic (or ongoing).

When it's acute, insomnia lasts for days or weeks, and it's often brought on by stress, worry, illness, hormonal shifts, environmental factors (such as noise), and the like. When it's chronic, it lasts for a month or longer and may be associated with chronic stress (like caring for a seriously ill family member or dealing with financial problems). Or it could be linked to an underlying medical problem such as allergies or asthma, reflux or chronic heartburn, an overactive thyroid, lupus, neurological diseases like Alzheimer's or Parkinson's, or chronic pain such as arthritis or back pain. Or it can stem from use of medications such as some that are taken for high blood pressure, heart disease, depression, or autoimmune diseases.

Insomnia is more common among women, and whether it's acute or chronic, the result is the same: We get too little sleep or poor-quality sleep and we wake up feeling tired, lethargic, foggy headed, depressed, or cranky. In fact, a 2014 study from Victoria University in Melbourne, Australia, found that women who reported sleep difficulties "often" in the year 2000 had more than double the risk of developing new-onset depression or anxiety in 2003, 2006, and 2009. What's more, insomnia can cause daytime sleepiness—which increases your risk of having an accident behind the wheel or while you're on your feet—and lessens your ability to focus, pay attention, learn new material, or remember important information.

Mild insomnia can often be treated effectively by improving sleep hygiene habits such as those previously described. For persistent, chronic insomnia that doesn't respond to these steps, it's best to see your doctor, who may recommend mind-body treatments such as cognitive behavioral therapy, which helps people clear their minds of thoughts that may cause difficulty sleeping; progressive muscle relaxation, which involves systematically tensing and then relaxing specific muscles in the body (often from head to toe); self-hypnosis; or deep breathing exercises—each of which can produce a state of physiological and mental relaxation that will help set the stage for sleep. Some people also benefit from sleep restriction therapy, which limits the time spent in bed to a specific number of hours, whether you sleep or not, in order to "reset" the body's natural sleep rhythm.

Many insomnia sufferers turn to over-the-counter sleep remedies—such as Unisom (doxylamine), Benadryl (diphenhydramine), or Tylenol PM (acetaminophen and diphenhydramine)—that contain an antihistamine. These are generally safe and fairly sedating. They can be useful as a one-off treatment for jet lag, for example, but they're not a long-term solution for sleep problems.

Another avenue that's better for treating chronic insomnia or poor sleep quality involves the use of natural sleep aids. For example, melatonin supplements—melatonin is a hormone that's made by the pineal gland in the brain and regulates sleep—can help restore your body's circadian rhythms and induce feelings of sleepiness when taken in the evening. Doses of melatonin supplements range from 0.2 to 20 milligrams; my recommendation is to start with a small dose and increase it as you feel you need to. Meanwhile, magnesium and calcium supplements have a calming effect on the body and mind, which aids sleep. I frequently use a product called Natural Calm, which contains calcium and magnesium in powder form (you simply add water and drink up); these minerals ease stress in the body and promote the release of calming neurotransmitters in the brain, a combination of effects that sets the stage for better sleep. Similarly, 5-HTP is an amino acid the body uses to make serotonin, a calming neurotransmitter that works to improve sleep quality; it's also available in supplement form.

In addition, soothing herbal aids such as chamomile or valerian tea (both of which are considered safe) induce relaxation and drowsiness. Other oral herbal sleep remedies that are popular (but haven't been studied extensively) include hops, passionflower, Jamaican dogwood, lemon balm, and Suntheanine (from L-theanine in green tea). One to skip: Kava kava, a root plant that is made into teas or supplements, is sometimes used to relieve anxiety or insomnia, but I recommend avoiding it because it can cause liver damage or even failure. Alternatively, you can harness the power of sleep-friendly scents like lavender, chamomile, ylang-ylang, jasmine, or vanilla with candles or by dabbing a few drops of essential oil on your pillow or applying a diluted version on the insides of your wrists and on your temples, all of which have been found to promote calm feelings that improve sleep.

The next step up on the sleep-inducing hierarchy is prescription sleep aids, such as Lunesta (eszopiclone), Sonata (zaleplon), Ambien (zolpidem), Rozerem (ramelteon), and Silenor (doxepin). These are generally short acting, which lowers the likelihood of feeling hung over the next morning. Most of these drugs make it easier to fall asleep, reducing the time it takes to enter the Land of Nod, while Silenor is useful for people who have trouble staying asleep. These drugs are not believed to be physically addictive, though psychological dependence often occurs. I recommend their use if the previous measures aren't working.

Other prescription medications used to treat insomnia include benzodiazepines, muscle relaxants, antidepressants, and other drugs. Benzodiazepines—such as Xanax (alprazolam), Ativan (lorazepam), Klonopin (clonazepam), Valium (diazepam), and Librium (chlordiazepoxide)—are a class of drugs used to treat significant anxiety and sometimes insomnia since they have sedating effects; in the latter respect, they are most useful for helping people fall asleep (they're not as effective with helping people *stay* asleep). They should be taken on a short-term basis only, due to the potential for patients to build tolerance or become addicted to them. Older antidepressants such as Desyrel (trazodone), Sinequan or Silenor (doxepin), and Elavil (amitriptyline)—as well as the newer antidepressant Remeron (mirtazapine)—are often used for insomnia because they relieve pain and cause sleepiness as a side effect. Pain medications such as Neurontin (gabapentin), Gabitril (tiagabine), and Lyrica (pregabalin) are also used as sleep aids because they're sedating and relieve pain, especially nerve pain. Muscle relaxants such as Soma (carisoprodol) and Flexeril (cyclobenzaprine) are occasionally prescribed for insomnia, but because of the potential for addiction and abuse, they're rarely the first-line choice.

As a last resort, antipsychotic medications such as Seroquel (quetiapine) and Zyprexa (olanzapine) are used to treat insomnia because they're very sedating; the downside is that they have a pretty significant side effect profile including daytime drowsiness, weight gain, abnormal heart-rate rhythms, and other unwanted symptoms. Years ago, barbiturates like phenobarbital, pentobarbital, and secobarbital were prescribed to treat anxiety and insomnia, but they've fallen out of favor because of their addictive potential and their propensity to produce withdrawal symptoms or rebound effects on REM sleep when they're stopped abruptly.

Depending on your personal circumstances, your doctor may suggest trying one of these drugs sooner or later in your quest for an insomnia remedy. But it's a mistake to rely on medications, supplements, or relaxation therapy alone. Each one of these interventions is more effective if you also practice good sleep hygiene habits. On the other hand, don't be afraid to work with your doctor and take medicine if you need it. Remember: The goal is to get a good night's sleep, night after night.

Sleep-disordered breathing: Many people take it for granted that they breathe normally while they're asleep, but this isn't always true. Sleep-disordered breathing occurs on a spectrum from loud snoring (which often occurs with allergies, colds, or congested sinus passages, or from consuming too much alcohol) to sleep apnea. Sleep apnea is a condition, affecting approximately 22 million people in the United States, in which the person periodically stops breathing for 10 seconds or longer while she sleeps. These breathing pauses may occur 30 times or more per hour. How frequently they occur determines whether sleep apnea is mild, moderate, or severe.

There are different forms of sleep apnea: obstructive sleep apnea, the most common type in which the airway collapses or becomes blocked during sleep, causes the person to resume breathing with a snort or choking sound; central sleep apnea, which occurs when the brain doesn't send proper signals to the muscles that control your breathing; and complex or mixed sleep apnea, a combination of the other two types. All three forms cause the sleeper to wake up multiple times—sometimes hundreds of times—during the night. During these mini-awakenings, the body senses poor respiration—loud snoring is often a sign of sleep apnea—and sends a signal to the brain to wake up just long enough to restore muscle tone and open the airways to help you take a proper breath. Usually the sleeper isn't aware of these pauses in breathing because they don't result in full awakening.

While sleep apnea is more common among men, the incidence rises in women after age 50, and the condition can occur in anyone at any age, even children. Obesity increases the risk of sleep apnea by obstructing the upper airway; in fact, 70 percent of people with obstructive sleep apnea are overweight or obese, according to the American Sleep Apnea Association. The condition is also more common among those who have a thicker neck circumference (which is often associated with a narrower airway), smokers, and those who have a family history of the disorder. Still, because of the lack of awareness among the public and even health-care professionals, the vast majority of people who have sleep apnea haven't been diagnosed and therefore remain untreated.

This is unfortunate, because aside from causing disrupted sleep and daytime sleepiness, this sleep disorder has serious consequences for your health, well-being, and functionality. If left untreated, sleep apnea can lead to high blood pressure, cardiovascular disease, stroke, diabetes, memory problems, depression, weight gain, impotence, and headaches. Moreover, untreated sleep apnea increases the risk of car crashes and work-related accidents or errors. If you suspect you have a form of sleep apnea, it's important to see your doctor, who may refer you to a sleep lab for a comprehensive overnight evaluation—called polysomnography—to examine your breathing patterns, other bodily functions, and brain signals while you're sleeping.

If you are found to have sleep apnea, several interventions can be beneficial. For those who are overweight, slimming down can improve the condition. In a 2014 study involving older adults with obstructive sleep apnea, researchers at Towson University found that participants who followed a weight-loss diet and exercised 3 days per week experienced improvements in the severity of their sleep apnea after 12 weeks, as well as a 9 percent drop in body weight, a 5 percent decrease in body fat, and a 20 percent improvement in aerobic capacity. Oral appliances, such as mouth guards that reposition the lower jaw to keep the airway open during sleep, decrease symptoms of mild sleep apnea. People with moderate to severe sleep apnea may be advised to use a breathing mask—the most common one is called a CPAP (continuous positive airway pressure) machine—that delivers a pressurized airflow into the sleeper's throat to prevent the airway from collapsing during sleep. For some people, surgery also may be an option.

One of my patients, a mother of two high school–age kids who was in her midforties, regularly slept 8 hours a night but remained exhausted. Her partner reported that she snored loudly, so I sent her for a sleep evaluation at a lab. The diagnosis: moderate sleep apnea, with more than 50 microawakenings at night. She tried the CPAP machine but couldn't tolerate it, so we began investigating other treatment options. She was discovered to have a benign cyst that was narrowing her airway during sleep; once it was removed, her sleep apnea improved greatly—and so did her exhaustion.

In my case, I also tried the CPAP machine, but it was so loud and disruptive that I couldn't tolerate it either, and I didn't notice a difference with a mouth guard. So I have learned to prop myself up on a bunch of pillows in bed at a 45-degree angle to help keep my airway open, and to sleep on my side as much as possible. Because my sleep apnea is quite mild, postural adjustments have helped me gain more restful sleep. With some trial and error, nearly every woman who suffers from sleep apnea can improve the quality of her sleep.

Restless legs syndrome: Another source of sleep disruptions, restless legs syndrome (RLS) is a neurological disorder that produces an irresistible urge to move your legs, resulting in microawakenings during sleep. More than 15 million adults in the United States suffer from it. Some people describe it as a creeping, crawling sensation; others experience it more as a tingling, throbbing, or burning feeling. Either way, moving the legs seems to make them feel better for a little while, but the pattern makes it hard to fall asleep or stay asleep. More than 80 percent of people with RLS also experience a condition called periodic limb movement disorder (PLMD), which causes periodic muscle twitches in the legs that may awaken the person from sleep.

In most cases, the cause of RLS remains a mystery, though there may be a genetic tendency toward the disorder. It can be brought on or aggravated by a condition (such as anemia, diabetes, or pregnancy) or a medication (like antinausea or antipsychotic drugs, antidepressants that increase serotonin levels, and cold or allergy medicines that contain sedating antihistamines).

There isn't a lab test for RLS. The condition is diagnosed based on a set of four criteria: Symptoms are worse at night and largely absent during the day; there's a strong, often overwhelming desire to move the legs; symptoms are triggered by sleep or rest; and symptoms are relieved by movement. Blood tests can reveal vitamin or mineral deficiencies (such as low iron, folate, magnesium, or B_{12}) or other medical conditions that are associated with RLS.

Lifestyle changes—such as reducing alcohol and caffeine consumption, quitting smoking, getting moderate exercise during the day, and doing relaxation and stretching techniques before bed—are often recommended to reduce symptoms of RLS and PLMD. If those don't work, medications (such as drugs that increase dopamine levels) may reduce symptoms. In addition, other drugs—such as benzodiazepines, opioids, anticonvulsants, and antipsychotics—are occasionally prescribed in an off-label capacity (this means that while these drugs are approved by the FDA for other conditions, they are sometimes used for RLS and PLMD, too).

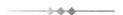

If you're skimping on sleep on a regular basis, or even if you're routinely spending a reasonable amount of time in bed and your sleep is simply not restorative, this is your wake-up call to take action. Sleep isn't an optional commodity, even in a 24/7 world. It's an indispensable ingredient in staying well, functioning optimally, having enough energy, curing exhaustion, and generally feeling good. Make it a point to carve out enough time for good-quality shut-eye—or to solve your sleep problem with the help of your doctor (and the fatigue diary in Appendix A). Your waking life really does depend on it.

The 411 on Sleep Cycles

Once upon a time, and not that long ago, it was believed that our brains and bodies shut down, almost like a computer, when we'd go to sleep. The thinking was that this passive state of rest would allow us to recover from the previous day and recharge for the next one. Now it's known that sleep is a lot more complicated than that.

The truth is, sleep is made up of five distinct stages, during which our brains and bodies experience various changes. Non-REM sleep consists of stages 1 to 4, each of which lasts from 5 to 25 minutes. This is when the body repairs and regenerates tissues, builds bone and muscle, and strengthens the immune system. A complete sleep cycle consists of a progression from stages 1 to 4 before REM (rapid eye movement) sleep occurs; then the cycle begins again. Here's how the stages play out.

- **STAGE 1**: As the person drifts off to sleep, muscle activity and eye movements slow down, but the sleeper can be easily awakened from this stage of sleep because it's so light. This stage typically lasts for 5 to 10 minutes before moving into . . .

- **STAGE 2**: During this period of light sleep, which lasts up to 25 minutes, there are brief increases in brain wave frequency before brain waves slow down. Meanwhile, the heart rate slows down and body temperature decreases as the body prepares to enter deep sleep.

- **STAGES 3 AND 4**: These are stages of deep sleep (aka slow-wave, or delta, sleep), which is more restful. Stage 4 is deeper and more restorative than stage 3. The brain becomes less responsive to outside stimuli, which is why it's more difficult to awaken a sleeper from this stage.

- **REM SLEEP**: Usually, REM sleep occurs 70 to 90 minutes after a person falls asleep. The first period of REM typically lasts 10 minutes, with each subsequent REM period lengthening; the final one may last up to an hour. In people without sleep disorders, heart rate and breathing speed up and the eyes move rapidly in different directions. Intense dreaming occurs during REM sleep as a result of heightened brain activity. REM sleep also plays an important role in learning and memory function, as this is when the brain consolidates and processes information from the previous day so that it can be stored in long-term memory.

If you're constantly being aroused from sleep, your body won't complete the four-stage non-REM sleep cycle. Instead, you'll be left in a repetitive cycle of stages 1 and 2, without reaching the critical, deep, restorative stages of 3 and 4. As people get older, we tend to sleep more lightly and get less deep sleep, but studies show the amount of sleep that's needed doesn't appear to diminish with age.

CHAPTER FOUR

Tired and Wired: Managing the Stress Factor

UNLESS YOU LIVE ON an ashram, stress is a fact of life in our modern world. Ask any busy woman whether she's under stress and the answer is likely to be: "Yeah, who *isn't*?!" Between perennial traffic jams, overbooked schedules, the dire economy, marital spats, rebellious children, and other sources of stress, most of us have plenty of factors that cause our shoulders to tense or our blood to boil. But we may not always be aware of the heavy toll that chronic stress exacts on our physical and psychological health.

The truth is, not all stress is created equal. There's acute stress like having someone try to swipe your purse or being cut off by an aggressive driver, and then there's chronic stress like taking care of a seriously ill family member or struggling to pay your bills month after month. There's good stress (which psychologists call eustress) such as getting married or moving to a new home; then there's bad stress such as having to deal with a difficult boss or disciplining a defiant or rebellious child. Good stress can be motivating, even invigorating, spurring you to strive to accomplish certain goals or rise to a worthy challenge. Positive stress sharpens our thinking, sparks our creativity, fires up our energy, and boosts our productivity. By contrast, bad stress, which is what most of us think of when we think of stress, tends to have subversive effects on the body and mind, essentially draining our energy and vitality.

The physiological effects of stress stem from a primitive but adaptive survival mechanism that dates back to the cavewoman era. At the first sign of a serious threat to our well-being, our bodies are primed for sudden movement in case we need to fend off a wild animal or run for our lives. That's when our bodies activate the fight-or-flight response: The hypothalamus in the brain triggers the release of stress hormones such as adrenaline and cortisol, which cause your breathing and heart rate to speed up, your blood pressure to rise, your eyes to dilate, and your muscles to contract. While this response is temporarily energizing and incredibly helpful if you need to fend off an attacker, it won't help you cope with a hot-tempered boss or other day-to-day stresses.

Unfortunately, nature wasn't planning for the less dire but chronic day-to-day stresses of modern living with this response. The body's stress-response program, which is activated by the neuroendocrine system's hypothalamic-pituitary-adrenal (HPA) axis, is supposed to be self-limiting. Once a perceived threat has passed, physiological functions should return to normal: The surge of adrenaline and cortisol that occurred should dissipate, your breathing and heart rate should slow down, and other bodily functions should get back to business as usual. But when stress is ongoing or prolonged or you constantly feel under siege, the stress response can stay turned on, sounding a continuous alarm in your body and mind.

The trouble is, when the stress response gets stuck in this "on" position, it can deplete your energy and take a toll on your body—from head to toe. This creates that running-on-empty feeling. Some health experts believe long-term stress leads to adrenal fatigue or adrenal burnout, which is obviously not good. Others attribute the exhaustion and feelings of general unwellness that occur with ongoing stress to the pervasive inflammation that high levels of stress hormones (like cortisol) cause throughout the body. The jury is still out on the exact mechanism, but it's widely recognized that fatigue is often a natural consequence of chronic stress.

Adding insult to lethargy, too much stress can also trigger digestive distress, headaches, hormonal imbalances and period problems, insomnia, heart palpitations, low sex drive, muscle pain, skin rebellions, a downturn in immune function (making you more susceptible to colds and infections), depression and anxiety, compromised cognitive function and memory impairment, and other unpleasant conditions. Women are more likely to report physical and emotional symptoms associated with stress, according to the 2010 American Psychological Association (APA) Stress in America survey. Chronic stress also has insidious long-term effects on the body. When the stress alarm goes off and doesn't shut off, the body's internal system of checks and balances—namely, its need to maintain homeostasis, a stable, steady internal state—is thrown out of whack. If a stressful situation goes on too long and the fight-or-flight response stays activated, this persistent state of being stressed out can cause physiological wear and tear to the body called allostatic load, the damage that results when the fight-or-flight response is functioning improperly.

Lifestyle habits (such as sleep deprivation, smoking, lack of exercise, and consuming an unhealthy diet or overeating) as well as certain states of mind (such as anticipatory anxiety) contribute to allostatic load. In his book *The End of Stress As We Know It,* Bruce McEwen, PhD, professor and head of the laboratory of neuroendocrinology at Rockefeller University in New York City, points out that besides occurring with unremitting stress, allostatic load may also happen when the body has an inappropriately intense response to stress that isn't lengthy or severe or when a person's body or mind doesn't hear the all-clear signal and shut off the fight-or-flight response after the stressful event has ended. Each of these scenarios triggers the release of high levels of stress hormones (such as adrenaline and cortisol), which may have harmful long-term effects on your body and mind.

Here's proof: In a study involving 104 female schoolteachers, researchers at the University of Trier in Germany found that chronic work stress was associated with both exhaustion and measures of allostatic load (such as elevated stress hormone levels, high blood pressure, cholesterol abnormalities, and elevated blood sugar). The physiological changes that occur with allostatic load can even speed up the aging process. A 2012 study, involving 2,911 women and men in Finland, investigated whether work-related exhaustion, a sign of prolonged work stress, is associated with accelerated biological aging, based on the length of telomeres (the protective caps at the ends of chromosomes). A bit of background: As people get older, their telomeres become increasingly damaged and shortened over time, which leads to DNA damage and an increased spiral of cellular aging. The study from Finland found that people with severe exhaustion had considerably shorter telomeres than their peers who weren't exhausted, which suggests that "work-related exhaustion is related to the acceleration of the rate of biological aging."

In the APA survey, women reported fatigue as a symptom of stress more often than men did; indeed, fatigue was the most common stress-related physical symptom women experienced. Stress can also affect your lifestyle habits, causing you to eat too much or indulge in junk foods, shirk your workouts, drink too much alcohol, smoke, or engage in other behaviors that could harm your health. Unfortunately, these reactions to stress create a vicious cycle—by depleting your body's natural stress-relieving defenses, they raise stress levels even more. In the Stress in America survey, women were 50 percent more likely than men to report eating as a way to manage stress, particularly eating too much or eating unhealthy foods—and while women said they wish they had more willpower to change their eating habits, they cited lack of energy or excessive fatigue as the primary barrier to improving their willpower. Moreover, sacrificing sleep, overloading yourself with caffeine, and consuming excessive amounts of alcohol can also elevate cortisol levels, thereby stimulating the HPA axis and exacerbating the body's stress response.

Nearly 50 percent of the women in the APA survey said their stress has increased over the last 5 years, with married women reporting higher stress levels than single women. This may result in part from the second shift that occurs for many women: the work women perform at home—taking care

Are You Experiencing Digital Drain?

There's no question that personal technology has made many aspects of our lives easier and more convenient—but this development comes with a cost: Living in a wired world that never fully shuts down contributes to stress. It's not just the 24/7 aspect of being constantly accessible by cell phone, text, and e-mail that's stressful, though that alone would be enough.

The constant exposure to the light on these devices stimulates brain activity, which is why checking your cell phone before bed can make it more difficult to doze off. Any electronic gadget's artificial blue light can suppress release of the sleep-inducing hormone melatonin. There's also the ever-present threat of the device ringing or dinging. A 2011 poll by the National Sleep Foundation found that 20 percent of people ages 19 to 29 are awakened by a call, text, or e-mail at least a few nights a week. Take this as a lesson: Be sure to power these gadgets down well before bedtime!

In addition, working on a laptop or a heavy handheld device for long periods of time leads to neck stiffness, headache, and fatigue. And checking your phone often may contribute to mental drain. Research suggests the average smartphone user checks her phone every $6\frac{1}{2}$ minutes, which adds up to approximately 150 times per day. Meanwhile, a 2012 study by McKinsey & Company found that high-skill knowledge workers spend 28 percent of their time reading and answering e-mail. Besides being disruptive, the frequent ping of e-mails landing in our in-boxes is stressful.

A psychiatrist I know suggests people put down all electronic devices for a period of time every 2 hours to give themselves a mental break from all this tech stress. This includes walking away from your computer for even brief periods throughout the workday. My recommendation is to also take regular e-mail vacations—by silencing or deactivating your mobile e-mail account for at least a few hours after work. Taking steps to protect yourself from digital drain will pay off mentally and physically.

of children, doing housework, preparing meals, and so on—after their paid workday is over. This double duty can be exhausting.

In a study involving 6,515 women born between 1960 and 1979, researchers at the Karolinska Institute in Stockholm, Sweden, analyzed self-reported health, fatigue, and symptoms of anxiety in relation to the participants' work status, work hours, and whether they had children or an employed partner. Employed women who had children reported the most fatigue and symptoms of poor health; the presence of a working partner buffered the effects only slightly. Another study from Sweden found that women are more likely to feel exhausted from high levels of work-to-family conflict and family-to-work conflict than men are. Job strain and low job support—which women suffer from more often in both cases—were also contributing factors.

Without a doubt, stress can have a far-reaching ripple effect on a woman's health and energy. In the context of fatigue, stress becomes almost viciously cyclical: Feeling wiped out or having too little energy to do what you want to do creates mental stress, and that further saps your energy. How you respond to stress is likely to be determined by a combination of genetic factors (some people have genes that predispose them to over- or underreact to stress) and life experiences (such as having experienced traumatic events in the past). It's important to remember that stress is in the eye of the beholder. What feels stressful to one woman may not be a big deal to another. Similarly, we all have our tipping points where the strain we're under can add up to serious overload, and those thresholds vary considerably from one person to another.

When my fatigue was so debilitating in medical school, several doctors blamed it on stress, saying things like, "Obviously it's the long hours you're keeping as a medical student." But I didn't buy this explanation. For one thing, after I would take a big exam or complete a major task, I would often feel a significant burst of energy (though it was usually short lived). I also never really felt stressed out by medical school in and of itself; I was more worried about whether I'd have the energy to get through it and be able to do everything I was supposed to do. In my case, I think my fatigue caused stress for me as much as the other way around.

While most of the women I see in my medical practice who complain of fatigue know if they're under stress, sometimes they don't realize the extent to which it's draining their energy. Take Monica, a 45-year-old single phlebotomist who worked four 12-hour shifts per week and was the sole care provider, physically and financially, for her aging parents. When I began treating her, her father had Alzheimer's disease and her mother was wheelchair dependent; she had recently moved them into her one-bedroom apartment, where she fed, bathed, and clothed them and tended to all their needs. Basically, she put her entire personal life on hold to care for them.

Monica was so exhausted that she began sleeping through the alarm and falling asleep in the break room at the hospital. She couldn't understand why this was happening, since she was sleeping at least 7 hours a night, so she asked me to check her thyroid. Her lab results were normal. I suggested that she learn relaxation and stress-relief techniques, but she said she didn't have the time or financial resources to do so; she did make an effort to ditch her fast-food habit and improve her diet, though. By her 1-year follow-up appointment, her energy had returned to normal, primarily because her stress level dropped considerably. Her father had passed away, and she moved her mother to a long-term care facility after the elderly woman suffered a near-fatal stroke. During the appointment, Monica told me she felt guilty admitting to herself how stressful her situation had been because she believed caring for her parents the way she did was "the right thing to do."

As with sleep, any efforts you make to reduce stress in your life or improve the way you handle it are likely to have a positive effect on your energy level. Unlike Monica's situation, many stressful experiences don't have a natural endpoint. That's why it's critical to make a conscious and deliberate effort to manage and reduce stress, even when you're up against seemingly impossible obstacles. To make yourself more stress resistant, strive to consume a healthy diet, exercise regularly, and get plenty of sleep. Also, make a point to spend time with valued friends, even when you're super-busy. Having supportive people in your life mitigates the effects of stress, allowing you to manage it more effectively, and makes you feel more resilient. (To our credit, women do a better job than men of staying connected to friends and family when we're stressed out, according to the APA's Stress in America survey.)

On a regular basis, try following these stress-relieving strategies.

Get moving. Exercise is one of the most effective stress relievers around. Simply taking a brisk walk, riding a bike, or participating in an aerobics class can decrease psychological distress, thanks to the release of endorphins and other feel-good neurotransmitters. Research from the University of Regina in Canada even found that doing aerobic exercise (in this case, riding a stationary bicycle) three times a week for 2 weeks significantly reduced post-traumatic stress disorder and anxiety sensitivity in those suffering from the disorder.

One of my patients, named Susan, is a stay-at-home mother of three teenagers. While in her early fifties and after being married for 20 years, she learned that her husband was having an affair. He didn't want to leave his mistress, but he didn't want a divorce (partly for financial reasons and partly so he could continue to live with his kids)—so he proposed having an "open" marriage. Susan didn't want this, but she didn't want a divorce either. As she was trying to decide what to do about this incredibly stressful situation, she began worrying "all day, every day" about the possible effects it could have on her, the kids, and their social life. She felt constantly tired but also wired with worry. An examination and a battery of lab tests revealed that she was in good health, and it became clear that the emotional exhaustion, anxiety, and stress she was going through were the basis of her fatigue. Because she was already seeing a therapist, I suggested she add regular exercise to her routine, which improved her energy level and eased some of the stress she was experiencing.

My Stress-Relieving Walking Rx

This is what I recommend as an antistress exercise prescription:

Start with 20-minute walks four times per week (on 3 weekdays, plus Saturday or Sunday). Walking is low enough in intensity that even if you feel overwhelmed, you're unlikely to feel like you don't have enough energy to get it done; it's also something you can do on your own schedule. Plus, even if you aim for just 20 minutes, often you'll stay out longer.

It's best if you can walk in a park or green environment so you can soak up some vitamin D from the sun and get the therapeutic value of time spent in nature. I recommend exercising in the morning, if possible, because studies suggest that morning exercisers are considerably less likely to cancel than those who save their routine for later in the day (when life has a way of throwing a wrench in the best-laid plans). Also, for antistress purposes, checking off the exercise box early in the day means you have one less thing to occupy your already overloaded mind.

Make a "to-don't" list. If your to-do list is constantly overwhelming and unrealistic—a sure sign is that you never get to the bottom of it and *that* stresses you out—it's time to do less. The best ways to do this are to learn to say no to nonessential requests, to delegate responsibilities to other family members or outside help, and to set limits with other people. If you've been a yes-woman in the past, it's time to do an about-face and start saying no.

The reality is, you only have so much time, energy, and attention to devote to various tasks and responsibilities in your life. Pick the ones that are essential, meaningful, or rewarding and make those a priority. Figure out what needs to be done today, what can wait until tomorrow, and what can be put off a bit longer. Using time-management strategies like these will save your sanity and reduce your stress. In the meantime, learn to pass up less appealing opportunities or tasks and cross them off your mental to-do list.

Give yourself regular time-outs. When you start to feel tension mounting in your body or mind, take a short break to hit the reset button. Find a quiet place at work or in your home where you can be alone and engage in a calming exercise—whether it's deep breathing, progressive muscle relaxation, visualizing a peaceful scene, listening to soothing tunes, or inhaling a calming scent (like lavender or vanilla)—for 3 to 5 minutes. Hopefully, you'll emerge from the break feeling refreshed and ready to refocus.

Calm your internal chaos. The goal is to establish a state of inner calm that enables you to stand up to stress and cope better with life's slings and arrows. Many different relaxation techniques can dial down your physiological and emotional reactivity to stress and restore an internal sense of calm. Indeed, regularly performing meditation, progressive muscle relaxation, tai chi, yoga, or repetitive prayer can ease the cumulative effects of stress on your body, research has found. Each of these relaxation techniques slows down your thinking and your brain waves as well as your blood pressure, your heart rate, and your breathing.

These changes relieve stress on the spot and leave you feeling more relaxed going forward, which counteracts some of the effects of stress over the long term. In a 2014 study at Kyushu University in Japan, 24 healthy women who had no experience with yoga underwent 12 weeks of yoga training and had their physical and psychological symptoms assessed before and after the training. By the end of the 12 weeks, the women scored significantly lower on measures of fatigue, anxiety, depression, and anger. Meanwhile, a 2014 study at the Indiana University School of Medicine found that a 7-week program of mindfulness meditation and yoga for persistently fatigued cancer survivors reduced the severity of their fatigue, allowed them to sleep better, and helped them gain enhanced vitality.

Put yourself in experts' hands. Acupuncture and cupping (an ancient technique in which cups are used to create suction on the skin to mobilize bloodflow and promote healing) are thousands-of-years-old approaches to stress management. Biofeedback and neurofeedback training teach you how to gain conscious control over unconscious bodily functions (such as heart rate, blood pressure, or brain wave patterns) that change in response to stress; these techniques are used most often to relieve stress-induced symptoms such as headaches, high blood pressure, sleep disorders, or chronic pain—but they can also calm your mind.

Change Your Mind to Change Your Stress

During my struggle with fatigue, I was particularly interested in whether stress was causing my exhaustion, or whether my exhaustion was making me feel stressed. With regard to the former, I noticed that when I was stressed about a major exam, my exhaustion was deafening, but as soon as the challenge was behind me, I felt a little (albeit short-lived) energy boost. So I spent some time educating myself about stress-reduction techniques and found that cognitive behavioral therapy (CBT) is one of the most researched and proven approaches. In particular, CBT is highly effective in treating anxiety disorders, including extreme stress, according to the National Institute of Mental Health.

The philosophy behind CBT is that it's not the events in our lives that cause stress but the way we think about them that induces the stress response in our bodies. So the therapy focuses on identifying and changing the way we think about and respond to challenging situations that feel stressful rather than trying to get rid of the stressors themselves. Learning to change your thought patterns takes practice, practice, and more practice— so you may benefit from working with a therapist who does CBT (fortunately, they're located all over the country).

In the meantime, try getting in the habit of giving your thoughts a makeover. After all, when you're under pressure or facing an intimidating challenge, it's easy to launch into forms of negative thinking that can actually exacerbate your stress. These patterns include catastrophizing (contemplating the worst possible outcome), all-or-nothing thinking (looking at things in black-and-white terms), jumping to conclusions (believing you know something to be true when your hunches could be seriously off base), and overgeneralizing (viewing a bad situation as part of an endless pattern of stress or bad luck).

To put matters in the proper perspective, try these strategies:

* Ask yourself how likely it is that your worst fears will actually happen.

* Consider whether the situation will really matter 3 months or 3 years from now.

* Banish words like *always* and *never* from your vocabulary and use kinder, gentler language to describe the situation you're facing.

* Question whether there's evidence to support your hunches or your assessment that a bad situation is part of a pattern or truly threatening.

In the course of standing up to your negative thoughts and reframing them, you'll probably discover that things aren't as dire as you initially thought and you will be able to relax a bit.

Consider what's within your control. When you are under stress and feeling powerless, it's easy and natural to focus on the upsetting things in your life that you can't control. But a better approach is to focus on what you *can* control. This strategy is called a cognitive flip. The idea is that when you feel powerless in a particular situation, you're able to curb your stress levels by paying attention to what you *can* control. To get a pulse on what those elements are, ask yourself what concrete steps, large or small, you need to take to improve a given situation or shape the outcome.

This technique helped one of my patients—Leah, who is a 40-year-old stay-at-home mom with two middle school–age children whose husband, a Wall Street executive, had lost his job in the recent financial crisis. Making matters worse, nearly all of their savings had been wiped out in the most infamous Ponzi scheme in US history—the Madoff investments. Her husband was spending most of his time following the crisis on the computer and was emotionally distant, so Leah single-handedly arranged to sell their apartment, relocate the family to a rental home in the suburbs, and enroll the kids in public school there.

Meanwhile, she tried to squelch the constant fatigue and stomach pains she was experiencing. She said she could barely muster the energy to take phone calls about important matters like trying to recoup their losses. Once an avid exerciser, she stopped completely when her husband lost his job. After putting her on medication for acid reflux, which had been exacerbated by her stress levels, I referred her to a therapist who focused on using cognitive behavioral therapy (CBT) to improve her ability to handle stress. Leah began doing deep breathing and other relaxation techniques regularly as well as practicing the cognitive flip: Instead of stressing about what she couldn't control, several times a day she would write down things she could control, like resuming her exercise regimen and being an attentive mother to her kids. Within a few weeks, she began feeling more empowered, and her energy level improved significantly.

Flick on the positive switch in your head. Instead of letting the stresses and strains in your life grab center stage, try to let the good things in your life take the spotlight—perhaps by making a list of specific things you're thankful for. The technique can bolster your mood, your mind-set, and your energy. Proof positive: When researchers at Arizona State University had people with rheumatoid arthritis keep diaries about their fatigue, their mood, and the number of positive and negative events that happened on a given day, women experienced decreased fatigue on the days when positive events outweighed negative events.

Ultimately, the best approach to reducing stress and reclaiming your energy is to put together a personalized toolbox of strategies that aid you. For me, that means making sure to exercise (yoga or power walking) 5 days a week, which relieves my shoulder pain and exhaustion. When life feels overwhelming (and it often does!), I make a concerted effort to stay in the present moment: I try not to play the "what if?" game. Instead, I focus on taking things one day at a time, even one period of the day at a time, to better pace myself. Improving the way I handle stress has increased my energy level, which in turn has lowered the amount of stress I experience. It's been a positive two-way street for me—I hope you can find your way onto it, too.

CHAPTER FIVE

Food Is Fuel: Eating and Drinking for Maximum Energy

FOOD REPRESENTS SO MANY different things to us that it's easy to overlook its essential purpose—as a source of fuel for our bodies and minds. It can still be a source of pleasure, a way to express love, a conduit for social connections, and more. But it's important not to lose sight of the fact that food provides the energy for your day-to-day performance. If you fill yourself with good-quality fuel, you'll increase your chances of having sufficient stamina, power, precision, concentration, and other qualities you value. If you don't eat enough or if you stuff yourself with junk food or convenience foods, you could wilt like a desert flower.

Unfortunately, many women fall into the latter categories. On a regular basis, I see patients and friends who engage in energy-sabotaging eating habits. They skip meals or fail to eat at regular intervals (often because they claim they're *too busy* to eat—but eating isn't optional; it's essential for survival). They consume too much or too little food at any given time, leading to calorie overload or the polar opposite (a calorie insufficiency). They skimp on key food groups—by not eating enough protein or healthy fats or by eliminating carbs, for example. They become extremely regimented and restrictive about what they will or won't eat, or they mentally obsess about what foods they will allow to cross their lips (a phenomenon researchers call cognitive dietary restraint, which has been linked with a higher excretion of cortisol—a sign of stress). Or they experience the flip side and regularly fall into food comas brought on by overeating or experience energy crashes after indulging in sugary treats. Or they shift from one hot fad diet to another and end up confusing their eating habits altogether. Each of these patterns takes a toll on your energy and vitality.

It's true that if you're overweight, losing weight is likely to improve your energy. This is partly because your body won't have to work as hard to tote around those extra pounds and thus it can free up energy for other activities. It's also partly because slimming down reduces elevated levels of systemic inflammation that can drain your energy. But if you're not trying to lose weight and you don't have intolerances or sensitivities to specific foods, there's no reason to cut out specific food groups or slash your calorie intake dramatically. If you do, you could end up sabotaging your own energy: Without enough nutrients from foods, you set yourself up for suboptimal cellular energy metabolism—the process through which food is converted to energy—which leaves you feeling tired, sluggish, and foggy. You could also develop suboptimal blood levels of certain nutrients, compromising your physical vim and vigor and your mental focus.

On the other hand, if you eat a lot of simple carbs, sugary foods, or processed foods, you'll likely experience rapid spikes in blood sugar and insulin, followed by a major blood sugar and energy drop along with carb cravings. Eat more carbs, and the roller coaster will begin its ascent (followed by another descent) again. It's a pattern that can make you feel utterly exhausted and cause a downturn in your metabolic rate. In a 2010 study at Pomona College, researchers compared the effects of consuming a sandwich made with a processed cheese product and white bread (processed foods) versus a sandwich made with multigrain bread and Cheddar cheese (whole foods) on posteating energy (or calorie) expenditure. Even though the two meals were comparable in terms of protein, carbohydrate, and fat composition, the processed-foods sandwich decreased the participants' postmeal energy expenditure by nearly

50 percent; besides having serious implications for potential weight gain, this after-lunch drop in metabolic rate will leave you feeling sluggish and tired.

My patient Tracy, a stay-at-home mother of two who's in her early forties, experienced this phenomenon firsthand. For years, she consumed a diet composed almost exclusively of fast foods and packaged snacks. While she did not consider herself obese or unhealthy—though she was both (she had high cholesterol, type 2 diabetes, and asthma, and her body mass index put her in the obese category)—she complained of severe fatigue. She spent her days watching TV and snoozing in her chair. During every visit, she would insist that her fatigue was what made her unable to change her eating and exercise habits, and she would often ask for blood tests to check for thyroid problems and other diseases that could cause fatigue.

For nearly 5 years, I tried to convince her to make dietary and other lifestyle changes, but she was disinterested in doing so—that is, until she was admitted to the hospital in hyperglycemic shock from poor diabetes control. She was in a medically induced coma for nearly a month and had two fingers amputated as a result of sepsis during the whole ordeal. After recovering, she gave up fast food, started a Weight Watchers program, and lost more than 100 pounds. She completely turned her lifestyle around—and her health!—and she is now full of energy.

THE ESSENTIAL PRINCIPLES OF EATING FOR ENERGY

For the sake of your energy and overall well-being, it's important to consume a diet based on nutrient-rich real foods with meals or snacks at regular intervals. Before I delve into the details of eating for energy, it helps to have a bit of biological background: All cells run on a high-energy compound called adenosine triphosphate (ATP), something your body basically uses like a battery to power various functions. (Biologists call ATP the energy currency of life.) ATP transports energy in cells, makes your muscles contract, and conducts nerve impulses, along with promoting other cellular processes. Food is a critical ingredient in this picture because ATP is obtained from the breakdown of food. Muscle cells manufacture ATP by combining the oxygen we breathe with nutrients we get from food, especially carbohydrates, although fat is sometimes used as well. When ATP is used up, it must be replenished from additional food and oxygen.

If you don't consume enough food and the right kinds of foods, you're essentially cheating your body of its prime power source. Food contains three main macronutrients—carbohydrates, fats, and proteins—and all are important for the production of ATP and muscle maintenance, among other bodily functions. Carbohydrates—which are present in grains, breads, pastas, rice, vegetables, fruits, legumes, and dairy products—provide a readily available source of energy for physical activity and the functioning of nearly every organ in your body. Fats—which are present in nuts, avocados, oils, fish, poultry, and meats—are needed to manufacture hormones and cell membranes, aid digestion, maintain skin health, and promote the absorption of fat-soluble vitamins. Proteins—which are found in eggs, certain grains, legumes, dairy products, fish, seafood, and meats—are important for the growth, repair, and maintenance of muscles and other tissues in the body.

With each of these macronutrients, it's important to choose the right types to optimize your energy and your health. This means consuming a variety of unrefined whole grains, vegetables, legumes, and fruits so that the nutrients and fiber in these foods remain intact—and avoiding processed or refined carbs, which lose most of their nutritional value. (Fiber is important because it's digested slowly, which helps maintain steady blood sugar levels and allows you to feel full for a longer period of time.) It means consuming enough monounsaturated and polyunsaturated fats, including omega-3 fatty acids, so your body will have the right stuff to carry out various functions (and avoiding artery-clogging saturated fats and trans fats). It means consuming enough lean protein so that you'll get the good-quality amino acids without excessive amounts of fat (and avoiding lots of red meat and full-fat dairy products).

In addition to supplying your body with energy, food provides your body with vitamins and minerals—these are called micronutrients—that play a critical role in helping the body function efficiently. Vitamins are chemical substances that naturally occur in various foods or are added to them (in fortified or enriched foods, for example); they are essential for the normal growth and development of cells, tissues, and organs and for various chemical reactions in the body (such as processing macronutrients from foods). Minerals come from the earth (especially rocks and metal ores), and we get these important micronutrients by eating plants that have absorbed minerals or by eating animals that have eaten the plants that contain the minerals; they play an important role in making and breaking down various body tissues (such as bone) and in regulating metabolism.

Here's the news you've been waiting for: A deficiency or even a suboptimal level of certain vitamins or minerals can lead to exhaustion, lethargy, concentration problems, and other unpleasant symptoms of depletion. While it's rare to see true nutrient deficiencies that are severe enough to show up on blood tests in healthy adults in the United States, there are a few exceptions in women: Vitamin B_{12} deficiencies frequently occur in those who follow a vegetarian diet; low iron levels (even iron-deficiency anemia) are seen in women with heavy menstrual periods and a low intake of animal protein and veggies; and vitamin D deficiencies are related to poor dietary intake, inadequate sun exposure, or both. All of these deficiencies (or insufficiencies) can lead to fatigue. (If you suspect you may be suffering from a deficiency, your doctor can make the diagnosis with a simple blood test.)

Similarly, if you don't consume enough carbohydrate, fat, or protein, you can lose steam quickly in your daily activities or you can feel as though you're running on empty—and essentially you are. That's because you haven't given your body enough of what it needs to function optimally or fuel itself sufficiently. Simply put, your body derives energy from the foods you eat or from its own internal energy stores; without enough of either (a readily available source of fuel or an ample fuel storage), your battery will run low and fatigue will set in.

If anyone knows this, it's my patient Barbara, a newly divorced lawyer in her early forties. She had always been diet and fitness conscious, but after her bitter divorce, she began to focus on "clean" eating. First, she eliminated all meat, dairy, and other animal products, then she cut out coffee, alcohol, and caffeinated tea; about a year later, she became strict about eliminating processed foods and artificial colors and flavors. She also worried about pesticides and the genetic modification of foods; every weekend, she was driving an hour and a half from her home in New York City to a farm in upstate New York to purchase vegetables that she believed had not been genetically altered. She had no social life because she felt she could not eat anything when she was out and about, not even in "vegan/health food" venues.

Even though she was very thin and had dry hair and nails, her blood work didn't indicate any nutritional deficiencies; yet Barbara complained of extreme fatigue during the day and an inability to sleep at night. After an extremely stressful job transition a year later, she finally agreed to some sessions with a therapist, which helped her ease some of her eating restrictions. I think it was the combination of consuming an extremely low-fat diet and the stress of being so regimented that was draining her energy. Once she relaxed her vigilance a bit, her mood and energy level gradually improved.

The Hidden Faces of Eating Disorders

Once considered the exclusive purview of teenage and college girls, eating disorders appear to be on the rise among adult women. It isn't known exactly how many of the 24 million people in the United States who are affected by eating disorders like anorexia nervosa, bulimia, binge-eating disorder, and ED-NOS (eating disorder not otherwise specified) are adults, but eating disorders experts say that in the last decade they've been seeing an increasing number of women over 30 who have disordered eating habits, if not full-blown eating disorders.

Some women who have eating disorders had them in adolescence and never got over them. Others seemed to recover, then the eating disorder made a comeback during a major life transition (like becoming a new mother or getting divorced) or a stressful period of time in their lives (like working in a toxic job environment). Meanwhile, other women engage in extreme behaviors—like weighing themselves excessively, obsessing about calories, abusing laxatives, and exercising to extremes—in an effort to preserve their youthful figures, prevent middle-aged spread, and forestall other aspects of the aging process. All of these patterns are energy-draining and lead to fatigue because they rob women of adequate nutrition and overload them with cognitive stress.

Then there's the relatively new phenomenon called orthorexia, an unhealthy obsession with eating healthfully. Eating "clean" (aka "organic") or eating "green" (as in sustainable or local) is frequently the goal. Often these folks won't let dairy products, wheat, red meat, sugar, salt, caffeine, alcohol, and other ingredients they consider unhealthy cross their lips. For many people, this healthy dietary pattern is empowering and gives them a sense of control—but it can be taken too far and can become obsessive, restrictive, or exclusive.

Usually, "orthorexia begins innocently enough," according to Steven Bratman, MD, author of *Health Food Junkies,* who coined the term in 1997. "But because it requires considerable willpower to adopt a diet [that] differs radically from the food habits of childhood and the surrounding culture . . . Most [people] must resort to an iron self-discipline bolstered by a hefty sense of superiority over those who eat junk food." Gradually, this pursuit can start to occupy a more significant proportion of the person's time and attention, and the pattern can become increasingly rigid. In my opinion, orthorexia crosses the line from healthy to unhealthy when it creates nutrient deficiencies, causes you to become underweight or fatigued, or negatively affects your social life and relationships. There's also a risk that such severely limited "healthy" eating regimens may serve as a bridge to anorexia or another point on the eating disorders spectrum.

Sticking with a healthy, energy-boosting diet isn't rocket science. It requires balance, moderation, and variety: a balanced intake of macro- and micronutrients, moderation in terms of portion size and calorie intake (especially for treats and desserts), and variety in terms of different foods within each category (grains, vegetables, fruit, legumes, nuts, fats, and lean protein). There isn't a particular diet that's guaranteed to crank up your energy. But in my opinion, the Mediterranean approach—which relies primarily on whole grains, vegetables, fruits, beans, nuts, legumes, and healthy oils (like olive oil) with smaller portions of fish and seafood, eggs, poultry, cheese, and yogurt, and occasional servings of red meat—hits the sweet spot for how to eat for optimal health and energy. I was a vegan for 9 years, until I took a trip to France and it became all about the cheese; now I eat dairy products in moderation as well as fish and chicken.

Heed the following guidelines and you'll be able to fill your plate or bowl with plenty of high-octane fuel.

Wake up your body with breakfast. Even if you're not hungry in the morning, having a morning meal kick-starts your metabolism and sends a signal to your body and your brain that it's time to perk up. It doesn't have to be a large meal, and you don't need to eat as soon as you wake up. But when you do eat, it's wise to have a combination of carbohydrates and protein: At the very least, have a piece of whole-grain toast with almond butter or a small bowl of whole-grain cereal with low-fat milk; if you're hungry, have a bigger meal such as quinoa topped with avocado and a poached egg, or a heaping bowl of oatmeal with bananas, raisins, walnuts, and cinnamon. The carbs will replenish your energy reserves and raise your blood sugar; the protein will increase alertness and provide feelings of lasting fullness—and the combination will set the stage for an efficient, productive morning. If you truly can't stomach the idea of eating breakfast, it probably means you ate too much the night before, a good habit to kick.

Mug Shot:
The Ups and Downs of Caffeine

When you're dead tired, caffeine can be an instant antidote, pepping you up and keeping you alert at crucial moments. A mild stimulant of the central nervous system, caffeine also revs up the heart, relaxes smooth muscles, increases stomach secretions, and has a diuretic effect. On the positive side of the ledger, caffeine can increase levels of neurotransmitters (brain chemicals) like norepinephrine, acetylcholine, dopamine, serotonin, epinephrine, and glutamate; these changes in turn increase alertness, attention, concentration, mood, and memory abilities and decrease fatigue. Caffeine can also give you a slight boost in metabolic rate, and regular caffeine consumption has been found to reduce the risks of Parkinson's disease and type 2 diabetes.

But caffeine becomes an energy-sapping substance when it's relied upon too heavily. It may increase blood pressure and cortisol secretion, cause shaky hands and anxiety, and contribute to insomnia and a delayed onset of sleep. Plus, if you're a java junkie who relies on caffeine (from coffee drinks, energy drinks and energy bars, and "natural" diet pills) to keep you going, the continuous rise and fall in stimulating effects is often accompanied by mild dehydration and symptoms of withdrawal—a bad combination.

It's a pattern that can lead to crashing and burning in the energy department. Believe me—I've been there! During my second year of medical school, when I was drinking a pot of coffee a day, I had built up such an extreme tolerance to caffeine that within an hour or two of having it, I would experience symptoms of withdrawal including fatigue, difficulty concentrating, and headaches.

When you get an energy boost after drinking coffee, it's not real energy—it's the effect of caffeine, a drug—and it's short lived. When the effects of caffeine wear off and your body realizes it doesn't have a true source of energy, you'll probably feel exhausted and maybe hungry. At that point, you might decide you need more caffeine, or you might choose to eat but end up overeating because you're in such a state of energy depletion. Either way, an unhealthy cycle begins again, one that can lead to a further energy drain.

The take-home message: Use caffeine wisely and pay attention to your total intake. Many women are fine with having coffee in the morning and then using caffeine occasionally as a temporary stimulant to increase alertness before an important meeting or before driving a long distance. If you find that you need additional pick-me-ups throughout the day, it's time to look at other energy-boosting measures (perhaps taking a brisk walk or a short nap, inhaling a whiff of a stimulating scent like peppermint, or splashing your face with cold water). Having more caffeine isn't the answer.

Eat regularly—and often. If you've been in the habit of eating erratically throughout the day, kick it. Instead, plan ahead and map out your meals and snacks so that you're eating something every 3 to 5 hours. Whether you opt for three square meals and two small snacks or five mini-meals spaced throughout the day is up to you. Either pattern will help keep your blood sugar steady and your energy level on a more even keel. (A hidden perk: You'll be able to benefit more often from the thermic effect of eating—the metabolic boost you get from digesting, processing, and storing food; this can help you burn 5 percent more calories per day, an extra 90 calories if you consume 1,800 per day.) To keep your energy and your metabolism revving high, it's important to consume enough calories each day. Don't skimp!

Eat real food only. Try to get the most nutritional bang for every bite by sticking with foods that offer a significant amount of nutrients for the calorie value—and come from identifiable sources. Good choices include vegetables, fruits, whole grains, beans and legumes, nuts, and seeds. Bad choices: refined breads, fried or fatty foods, sweets, desserts, and processed snack foods, all of which provide you with lots of calories but little in the way of nutritional value.

How Many Calories Do You Really Need?

There's an easy way to figure this out, based on the Harris-Benedict equation, which is used to estimate an individual's basal metabolic rate (BMR). Pull out your calculator or a pencil and paper and get ready to do some math.

1. Start with a base of 655 calories.

2. Multiply your weight (in pounds) by 4.3.

3. Multiply your height (in inches) by 4.7.

4. Add together these first three numbers and put this sum aside for the moment.

5. Next, multiply your age by 4.7.

6. Subtract the number from step 5 from the previous sum (step 4).

7. Now multiply the previous total (step 6) by the following, based on your physical activity levels:

   1.2 if you're sedentary (meaning you get little to no exercise)

   1.3 if you get light exercise (as in 2 to 3 hours per week)

   1.4 if you engage in moderate physical activity (approximately 4 to 7 hours per week)

   1.6 if you do high levels of physical activity (more than 7 hours per week)

The sum you end up with reflects the number of calories you need to consume per day to keep your weight steady and your body functioning well.

A good rule of thumb: If it comes in a box and lasts for a year, you'd be better off with something that was recently alive (as in fruits, vegetables, and whole grains). Similarly, if there are ingredients that you can't pronounce or recognize listed on the label of a packaged food, you probably don't want to be putting that item into your body. You need real food for real energy!

Put color on your side. Brightly hued fruits and vegetables—such as tomatoes, strawberries, carrots, sweet potatoes, oranges, yellow squash, broccoli, kiwifruit, kale, spinach, bell peppers, blueberries, eggplant, leafy greens, and others—are loaded with antioxidants that neutralize damaging chemicals called free radicals. These unstable molecules can injure cells, laying the foundation for a host of illnesses, disorders, or diseases to develop; antioxidants prevent or fight these detrimental effects while also boosting immune function. An inside tip: There's actually a way to measure the antioxidant levels in foods—it's called the ORAC value (short for Oxygen Radical Absorbance Capacity value). You can look it up (oracvalues.com) and see how your favorite foods, herbs, and spices rank.

To Juice or Not to Juice?

Unlike many traditional medical practitioners, I'm not entirely against juice fasts. But it's critical to keep the fanatical claims in perspective—and really understand what the fasts will do for you, and what they won't. The basics: A juice fast involves limiting your diet to *only* fresh fruit juices and vegetable juices, plus water, for a few days or longer. Supporters of the practice claim that juicing "detoxifies" the body, helps with weight loss, and prevents everything from the common cold to autoimmune diseases to various forms of cancer.

Over the years, I have done a number of different juice fasts. My most positive experiences have been with short 2- to 3-day vegetable-juice fasts. *(Who knew I could consume so many pounds of kale?!)* During the fast and for a week or so afterward, I find that I experience fewer cravings for greasy, salty, and fatty foods (suddenly fries are much less appetizing, and cheeseburgers look like dog food). I also sleep more soundly and feel a bit more energized, as if I've increased my vitamin intake by 4,000 percent (even though I really haven't).

But there are downsides. Juice fasts or cleanses are dangerous for some. People with diabetes can experience extremely high blood sugar from large amounts of fruit juice, and people who are on chemotherapy or who have kidney disease may suffer potentially life-threatening electrolyte imbalances. Juice fasts won't help you lose weight—or keep it off, if you do happen to drop a few pounds. And there's no scientific evidence to show that "detoxing" is beneficial for preventing any illnesses; the truth is, our liver, kidneys, and intestines detoxify our bodies naturally every day.

If you want to try a juice fast, avoid extremely restrictive versions (like the Master Cleanse), and don't stay on any juice fast for longer than 3 or 4 days. Focus on fresh fruit and veggie juices that you squeeze yourself, or purchase freshly made juices that haven't been pasteurized. While pasteurization kills potentially harmful bacteria, it also kills good microorganisms and decreases levels of some vitamins and minerals. To get the biggest nutritional boost from a juice fast, the fresher the juice is, the better it is for you.

Harness omega-3 power. Omega-3 essential fatty acids—which are plentiful in fatty fish (like salmon, halibut, tuna, lake trout, sardines, and anchovies) as well as flaxseeds, walnuts, canola oil, and fortified foods—reduce harmful inflammation throughout the body, protect the function and integrity of cell membranes, and enhance brain function. Research suggests that regular consumption of omega-3 fatty acids boost mood, memory, and other measures of cognitive function, which can boost your focus and energy. Try to include these food sources on a daily basis.

Give yourself permission to snack. If it's done right, snacking between meals keeps your mood and energy level on an even keel, fills in nutritional gaps in your diet, better regulates your appetite, and enhances your weight-control efforts. It'll also prevent overeating (which could leave you in a food coma) at your next meal. The key is to plan your snacks ahead of time—ideally, a combination of protein and carbohydrates—in a 200- to 300-calorie portion so you'll be less likely to give in to the siren call of the vending machine or the snack rack at a convenience store or newsstand when hunger strikes.

Don't make the mistake of equating *snacks* with (sweet or salty) *treats*. Snacks should consist of good-quality, nutrient-rich calories. Combining complex carbs with protein and healthy fat will provide a slower, more sustained rise in blood sugar, giving you lasting energy and feelings of fullness. Good choices include hummus with baby carrots and snap peas, low-fat plain yogurt with whole blueberries, whole-grain crackers with peanut butter, or a mix of nuts and dried fruit.

Drink H_2O as if your life depends on it. It actually does! Water accounts for approximately 60 percent of an adult's body weight. The human body has no way to store water, so we need to constantly replenish the fluids we lose through breathing, urinating, sweating, and other bodily functions. Believe it or not, many people are walking around in a mild state of dehydration, which may be contributing to why they feel tired, weak, or lethargic. In fact, a recent study in the *Journal of Nutrition* found that when women were put into a very slight state of dehydration—1 percent lower than optimal—with exercise and/or a diuretic drug, they experienced a sense of fatigue, low mood, headaches, and loss of focus during rest and during exercise. This is probably because when you're dehydrated, the fluid loss from your body causes a drop in blood volume, which makes your heart have to work harder to push oxygen and nutrients through the bloodstream to your brain, skin, and muscles.

Thirst is not a good indicator of your hydration status: Some data suggest that by the time you feel thirsty, you've already lost 2 to 3 percent of your body fluids. If you're dehydrated, you might actually feel fatigued before you feel thirsty. That's why it's important to plan out how you're going to drink just as you plan your meals. Get in the habit of carrying a water bottle with you and

A Drink to Your Health–Or Not?

Even though people tend to think of alcohol as a calming drug, those who are suffering from fatigue might actually experience a short energy boost after a glass of wine or a cocktail. But the next day, it will leave you more tired than if you had stuck with water. Here's why: For one thing, alcohol is a depressant, which means it can take a toll on your mood and lead to low energy. For another, while having a drink may make it easier to fall asleep, as your body continues to metabolize the alcohol, its latent stimulating properties kick in, paradoxically increasing the number of times you wake up, thus fragmenting your sleep. It also prevents you from getting enough deep sleep and REM sleep by keeping you in the lightest sleep stages.

Plus, alcohol has a dehydrating effect. Simply put, the process of metabolizing alcohol is dehydrating to the body. Hangover symptoms are mostly related to extreme dehydration. But even if you don't drink to the point of a hangover, just being slightly less well hydrated may leave you wiped out the next day: Along with thirst, one of the biggest symptoms of dehydration is fatigue. To prevent this from happening, it's best to limit your alcohol intake to no more than a drink or two per day—for a maximum of seven drinks per week—and to drink at least one glass of water between glasses of wine and cocktails.

refill it regularly throughout the day so that you consume eight 8-ounce cups of water per day. To make plain H_2O more exciting, you can add lemon or orange wedges or cucumber slices. You can also increase your water intake by eating fresh fruits and vegetables and soups. There's no need to drink vitamin waters or energy drinks unless you're an endurance athlete; otherwise, you're just adding unnecessary calories (and an unnecessary expense) to your day.

ENERGY-BOOSTING SUPERFOODS

You've probably heard the term *superfoods*—it's often applied to things like brown rice, spinach, yogurt, tomatoes, and other healthy fare—but have you ever wondered what makes a food *super*? It's not about taste, but taste does matter. It's really about efficiency: Superfoods not only pack more nutritional punch per bite than other foods do, they also have other properties that directly support the immune system, cut down on inflammation in the body, support mental health, and boost energy, stamina, and longevity. You can't ask for much more than that from a single food!

But here's a reality check: No food is super unless it tastes good, too, because otherwise you wouldn't be willing to eat it. With that in mind, here's my top 10 list of energy-boosting superfoods that everyone should eat on a regular basis.

Oats: These are arguably the most perfect superfood because they're high in fiber, protein, potassium, magnesium, and other minerals. Oats are best eaten at breakfast, because the fiber they contain is digested slowly, which stabilizes blood sugar levels all day. Oats have been shown in large-scale studies to lower cholesterol, which is why they're considered a heart-healthy food. If you're not a fan of oatmeal (I confess: I don't care for it), you can sprinkle them onto a bowl of cold cereal or yogurt, sneak oats into turkey meat loaf, or toss them into salads or casseroles for a nutritional boost.

Quinoa: This gluten-free grain has more protein than any other grain or rice. It's so rich in amino acids (such as lysine, cysteine, and methionine) that it's actually considered a complete protein (generally, complete proteins are only found in animal products). The amino acids help with muscle repair after exercise, while the folate, magnesium, and phosphorus in quinoa support energy levels.

Blueberries: In addition to being loaded with powerful antioxidants and energy-boosting carbs, blueberries contain vitamins A and C, folate, potassium, magnesium, and fiber. Research suggests that these nutrients, along with the phytochemicals (health-promoting compounds that give plants their pigment) in blueberries, boost immune function and lower depressive symptoms by stopping the buildup of free radicals. This helps the body and mind recover from stress and cellular injury faster.

Salmon: Loaded with anti-inflammatory omega-3 fatty acids (in particular, docosahexaenoic acid, or DHA, and eicosapentaenoic acid, or EPA) that improve heart health, salmon is also a stellar source of protein. The American Heart Association recommends having fatty fish like salmon at least twice a week. Dietary intakes of fish and omega-3 fatty acids have been found to reduce depressive symptoms and improve cognitive function. Salmon's energy-boosting effects are related to improved metabolism, including the more efficient use of oxygen in the body during exercise.

Avocados: A source of healthy fats, avocados are full of fiber, potassium, vitamins A and E, and folate. They're also a good source of an omega-3 fatty acid called alpha-linolenic acid, which improves the metabolic aspects of heart health including levels of oxidative risk factors, blood fat levels, and inflammatory markers (like homocysteine, which is often elevated in fatigue-causing conditions like diabetes, arthritis, and chronic fatigue syndrome).

Turkey: Not only is it low in fat and a good source of protein, but turkey contains the amino acid tyrosine, which elevates levels of dopamine and norepinephrine, brain chemicals that keep you more alert and focused. (Don't worry that eating turkey will make you sleepy because of its tryptophan; turkey doesn't have much more of this amino acid than chicken or fish does.) It also contains vitamins B_6 and B_{12}, which have been shown to ease insomnia and depression and boost energy.

Goji berries: Used for 5,000 years in Chinese medicine to stimulate energy and mental acuity as well as lower stress, goji berries are believed to increase bloodflow, causing energy-enhancing oxygen to flow more freely throughout the body. These bright orange-red berries are concentrated sources of antioxidants; they can be eaten raw, cooked, or dried like raisins.

Almonds: Packed with protein and fiber, almonds also contain calcium, potassium, phosphorus, and vitamin E. What's more, they're a rich source of magnesium, which plays a key role in converting sugar into energy. Having low levels of magnesium in your body can drain your energy and cause sleep problems and leg cramps.

Lentils: These legumes are powerhouse sources of low-fat protein, fiber, iron, potassium, zinc, and folate. They're also rich in selenium, a mineral that may be a natural mood enhancer; studies have linked low selenium levels to poorer moods and lower energy levels. The fiber in these petite legumes stabilizes blood sugar.

Kale: Loaded with vitamin C, vitamin A, calcium, iron, and potassium, this leafy green vegetable is also a solid source of protein and fiber—and it's very low in calories. In addition, it's packed with flavonoids, phytochemicals with antioxidant properties, which is why kale earns one of the highest ORAC ratings among vegetables.

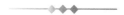

The link between what you eat and how your body and mind feel and function on any given day is indisputable. I can't emphasize enough that what you put into your body is what you get out of it, in terms of energy—so choose your foods wisely! There isn't a single approach to eating that maximizes energy for everyone, so you'll need to discover the winning food formula that works for you (in Chapter 14, you'll learn more about how to do that). This may require a bit of trial and error, but if you stick with real health-promoting foods, the right mix of nutrients, and a consistent eating pattern, it won't take long for you to find the best sources of edible energy that fuel your body and please your tastebuds, too.

CHAPTER SIX

Revving Your Engine: Finding Exercise That's Right for You

WHEN YOU'RE ALREADY EXHAUSTED, exercise may be the last thing you feel like doing. Indeed, a lot of people think they're doing themselves a favor by not exerting themselves physically if or when they're exhausted. But exercise could actually help rejuvenate you in the short term and stimulate your energy in the long term. Granted, the notion that expending energy through exercise could enhance your energy seems counterintuitive, but it makes good sense from a physiological perspective.

After all, spending long hours in a statuelike position in front of your desk or being sedentary in your free time can make you feel tired because your body equates stillness with sleep (or a desire to go to sleep). When you're sitting still, your breathing and heart rates slow down; your circulation does, too, bringing less oxygen and fewer nutrients to your brain and body tissues. Your muscles stop contracting, and your metabolism gets dialed down. Before you know it, you're yawning and fighting the urge to nod off.

On the other hand, shortly after you begin moving briskly, your heart rate and breathing rate will increase, your body temperature will rise, and your blood will flow more quickly, bringing vital oxygen and nutrients to cells throughout your body. Your muscles will contract, generating power and heat, which is essentially a form of mechanical energy inside your body.

Your metabolism will get revved up, too, which in turn boosts your circulation even more and allows more oxygen to reach your brain and muscles, thereby enhancing your energy level. On a cellular level, exercise increases the number of mitochondria, the energy sources—or batteries, if you will—inside cells, thus improving your body's ability to produce energy. (Being sedentary, by contrast, can cause a decline in mitochondria; the aging process can, too.) The more often you perform aerobic exercise, the more mitochondria your body will make, which will generate more energy during the exercise session and afterward.

Over time, aerobic exercise increases your consumption of oxygen and increases your lung capacity. As you get fitter, these changes lead to increased stroke volume—this means the heart beats more slowly and powerfully with each pump—which gives you greater stamina and endurance for exercising, playing sports, and performing everyday activities. As your lung capacity and cardiovascular fitness improve, you'll experience a more efficient delivery of oxygen to your brain and bloodstream, which can help you feel more alert, energized, and ready to go.

Plus, exercise is one of the most potent mood boosters around, thanks to the release of feel-good neurotransmitters such as serotonin and endorphins. These natural opioid-like chemicals are produced by the pituitary gland in the brain, and they can relieve pain and enhance well-being as they course through your bloodstream. In fact, when runners refer to the "runners' high," they're talking about the feelings of euphoria and energy they experience during prolonged, strenuous exercise, thanks to the release of endorphins into the bloodstream. But even moderate or light physical activity will cause your body to release some endorphins, creating similar, if not as strong, effects on your mood and energy level.

These effects don't even include the long-term health perks. The fact is, exercise has a laundry list of health benefits ranging from improved cardiovascular, pulmonary, and endocrine functioning to slowing down age-related cognitive decline and alleviating depression. Regular physical activity has been found to reduce the risks of developing cardiovascular disease, type 2 diabetes, hypertension, breast and colon cancer, osteoporosis, and many other life-threatening diseases. Increasing your level of physical activity, especially if you also make healthy dietary changes, can even reverse conditions such as type 2 diabetes and hypertension, as countless studies have shown and as I have seen in my own practice. Exercise also makes it easier to control your weight, which in turn relieves fatigue.

One of my patients, Kristen, is a 37-year-old newspaper reporter who works unpredictable hours, including many late nights followed by early-morning wake-up calls. Four years after having her first child, she hadn't been able to shed 15 pounds of baby weight she was still carrying, and she consistently felt wiped out. Even when her work hours were less frenetic, she felt like she couldn't get her sleep back on schedule; more often than not, she slept poorly with frequent awakenings. Her diet was healthy, but she wasn't getting any exercise, in part because she's not a "gym person" and doesn't like the atmosphere at health clubs.

I suggested she try another venue that would be more appealing to her, so she started doing 90-minute Ashtanga yoga classes four times a week in the morning. Within 2 months, she felt as if her life had been "transformed": She lost 10 pounds, began sleeping deeply and soundly, and began feeling energized throughout the day. Exercise produced a total turnaround for her.

Moreover, exercise is beneficial for your brain function and your mood. It enhances the flow of blood, oxygen, and nutrients to the brain and reduces the risk of Alzheimer's and other forms of dementia. More immediately, it improves attention, concentration, learning, and memory, which can boost your productivity. Regular aerobic exercise also eases anxiety and depression. In fact, researchers at Duke University found that aerobic exercise is as effective as antidepressants in treating major depression and preventing a recurrence.

What's more, recent research suggests that sitting still for long hours each day can shorten your life span: In a 2014 study involving 71,363 men and women ages 18 to 99, researchers in Denmark found that those who sit 10 or more hours per day and are physically inactive in their leisure time have more than double the risk of dying prematurely over a 5-year follow-up period than those who sit for less than 6 hours per day and are physically active in their spare time. If ever there were incentive to move more, enhancing your longevity—or preventing premature death—should be high on the list. If you work in a sedentary environment, I recommend getting up at least every 30 minutes to walk around, stretch, visit with colleagues at the water cooler, or find any way to get yourself moving again.

THE ENERGY-BOOSTING EXERCISE PRESCRIPTION

Here's the good news: You don't have to run marathons or compete in tennis tournaments to boost your energy. In most cases, a mild to moderate workout (such as a 30-minute brisk walk, an aerobics class, or a swim) lessens exhaustion by prompting the energy-producing mitochondria in your cells to ratchet up their activity. You'll also enhance your circulation, which in turn can raise your vim and vigor.

The exercise doesn't even need to be as strenuous as you may think to reap energy-boosting benefits. In a study involving 36 young adults who reported persistent feelings of fatigue, researchers at the University of Georgia randomly assigned the participants to a low-intensity aerobic exercise program, a moderate-intensity one, or a control group. After 6 weeks of three-times-a-week workouts, both exercise groups experienced improvements in their energy levels, while the low-intensity group reported more positive changes in their symptoms of fatigue than the moderate-intensity group did (both fared better than the control group). A subsequent study by the same researchers found that single sessions of low- and moderate-intensity exercise (in this case, cycling) enhanced feelings of vigor; again, fatigue improved more after the low-intensity sessions. My belief is if you're already tired, you're better off starting with low-intensity exercise to try to boost your energy rather than pushing your limits and risk depleting your energy reserves even more. Strength training can help as well: In another study, researchers from the University of Georgia found that when persistently tired, sedentary women performed moderate- to high-intensity resistance exercise (four sets of 10 repetitions of lower-body resistance exercises), they experienced increased energy during and after their workouts.

The challenge is to figure out the type and amount of exercise that is going to kick-start your energy and guide you toward your fitness goals. Starting with more enjoyable, less strenuous activities like walking, yoga, biking, swimming, and tai chi is ideal; this way, you'll look forward to the sessions and you'll be able to stop well before you get tuckered out. People with fatigue-related illnesses, including chronic fatigue syndrome and fibromyalgia, may feel worse after exercising—but often that's because they've pushed themselves too long or too hard. In most cases, a mild to moderate workout can contribute to relieving exhaustion associated with these conditions.

This is what a 30-something patient named Suzanne, a human resources executive for an insurance company, discovered. She was diagnosed with chronic fatigue syndrome (CFS) 2 years before our first visit, and when she came to see me, she was complaining of having relentless exhaustion, bouts of falling asleep at her desk, and nonrestorative sleep at night. Suzanne would often concoct excuses to miss morning meetings at work so she could sleep in for 3 more hours, but even this strategy didn't make her feel better. She had spent a fair amount of time improving her diet to combat CFS—eating frequent, nutrient-rich meals and avoiding foods she was sensitive to—and she used good sleep hygiene techniques and some herbal approaches, but she still didn't get relief from her fatigue.

Ironically, her husband worked as a personal trainer, but Suzanne said she didn't have the energy to exercise. I suggested she simply try walking at

Kinder, Gentler Mind-Body Exercises

A number of exercises that originated in Eastern cultures offer many of the same physiological and psychological benefits as more hard-core workouts—and they're believed to stimulate the body's inherent energy channels. Yoga, tai chi, and qigong (aka chi gong) provide gentle ways of building muscle strength and improving flexibility, balance, and coordination while also relieving stress. Each of these approaches relies on breath work, meditation, specific postures, and slow, fluid movements to stimulate the release and flow of the body's inherent energy (chi).

The underlying theory behind these modalities is that when the flow of the body's energy is blocked, it takes a toll on our health, our energy, and our overall sense of well-being. Stress is often to blame for these energy blockages, but other factors (including the aging process) contribute, too. The belief is that by engaging in gentle, fluid movements and specific breathing patterns, energy flow within the body is restored and a sense of greater health and well-being is achieved. It might help to think of these techniques as ways of harnessing the body's internal energy to stimulate the energy you want to use externally in everyday life. You can learn them at boutique studios and mind-body centers near you, or try a DVD that walks you through the basics.

Research has found that these techniques even help people with serious medical conditions improve their energy. In a 2014 study, researchers at the Ohio State University found that breast cancer survivors who participated in a 12-week program of 90-minute hatha yoga classes twice a week experienced reductions in fatigue, increases in measures of vitality, and lower markers of inflammation. Similarly, a 2014 study at Arizona State University found that breast cancer survivors who learned a meditative movement practice based on qigong/tai chi over 12 weeks showed significant improvements in measures of fatigue. And a study from Tufts-New England Medical Center in Boston found that 12 weeks of tai chi improved pain and vitality in adults with rheumatoid arthritis. Feeling really is believing!

a comfortable pace for 30 minutes five times a week to see if that would help. After 6 weeks, she reported feeling 50 percent less fatigue during the day—it was the biggest improvement any intervention had made to her condition.

If you've been sedentary until now, simply incorporating more movement into your days will boost your energy. Think of it as expending energy to produce more energy. Our bodies were made to move, and whenever we get moving, the physiological changes our bodies experience will generate more energy from the inside out. Starting an exercise routine doesn't have to be cumbersome; there are so many different ways of approaching physical activity that surely you can find one that suits your preferences. It may just take a little experimentation, perhaps even some trial and error, to find the fitness fit that works for you. Here are eight strategies to keep in mind as you embark on that discovery process.

Do what you like. If you enjoy walking or cycling outside, do that instead of going to the gym to use a treadmill or stationary bike. If you don't like taking aerobics classes at the gym, opt for an exercise DVD you can use at home or simply play your favorite tunes and dance, jump, and hop to your heart's content. If you love to swim, find a pool where you can do laps year-round. If playing competitive sports is more your speed, join a tennis, racquetball, volleyball, or softball league.

Schedule your workouts. Don't take a chance that last-minute requests or unexpected events will get in the way of your exercise time. Write your workout times into your calendar—whether you use a paper one or your smartphone—and treat them as sacred, as if they were important business or doctors' appointments. Research suggests that one of the best ways to ensure that you stick with your exercise program is to work out first thing in the morning, before any surprises have a chance to interfere with your good intentions.

Use exercise as your personal time-out. Your workout provides a natural break—the antidote, really—from the stresses of the day, so appreciate your movement time. Don't let other commitments get in the way or multitask by catching up on phone calls during your power walk, for example. Instead, clear your mind and let your thoughts wander; pay attention to the sights, sounds, and smells around you; or listen to enjoyable music on your iPod. Finding ways to make your workout pleasant will rejuvenate your mind along with your body.

Give Yourself Breathing Lessons

Breathing is such an automatic function that most of us don't give it a thought. But if you've ever noticed exercisers at the gym huffing and puffing in funky ways during a cardio workout or people who seem to hold their breath and then exhale dramatically while lifting weights, you may have wondered what constitutes proper breathing during exercise. The reality is, smooth, efficient breathing is vital for the delivery of blood, oxygen, and nutrients to muscles, organs, and other tissues throughout your body at any time, but especially during a workout. So it's important to do it right.

While the pattern of breathing in through your nose and out through your mouth can be beneficial during mild forms of exercise and mind-body workouts like yoga—since this pattern has a calming effect—it's often difficult to sustain this during more intense activity. When you're running or playing a high-intensity sport, for example, you'd be better off breathing deeply (from the diaphragm, not the chest) through your mouth. While lifting weights, by contrast, fitness experts usually recommend taking a few deep breaths to start, then exhaling through your mouth as you lift the weight and inhaling through your nose as you lower it. Whatever activity you're doing, it's a mistake to pant or hold your breath: These are inefficient ways of breathing that can increase fatigue, drain your energy, and impair your performance.

Slip in more movement. If you don't have time for a full-fledged workout, don't ditch your plans entirely. Go for a 10-minute walk during your lunch break or in the late afternoon. Do strength-training exercises (such as squats, lunges, and triceps dips) while you watch TV. Physical activity doesn't have to be an all-or-nothing proposition.

Find a fitness friend. If you find an exercise buddy—with whom you can work out at the gym or walk outdoors—you'll make physical activity social, which will likely make it more enjoyable. You'll also increase the odds that you'll adhere to the program you've set for yourself because you won't want to let your workout partner down. Instead, you'll keep each other accountable.

Embrace an energizing mantra. Find or come up with a statement or verbal cue that motivates you to get moving and maintain a positive state of mind. It could be something as simple as "Turn it on!" or "I'm getting stronger every day." What's most important is that it speaks to you in a way that encourages you to give your workouts your best effort, whatever that means for you on any given day.

Let your environment support your goals. Before you turn in for the night, pack your gym bag and put it by the front door. Or place your walking or jogging clothes and shoes by the side of your bed so you can step into them as soon as you wake up. Having your workout gear handy takes the guesswork out of having to find it—and serves as a visual reminder of what you plan to do.

Tune in to the feel-good rewards. Regularly pause and take note of how your workouts help you feel reinvigorated in the afternoon or kickstart your energy in the morning. Or how they boost your mood or clear the fogginess from your head. Pay attention to how much sounder you sleep or how much better regulated your appetite is. Focusing on these energy- and health-related results provides built-in motivation to keep up the good work.

RESPECTING THE EXERCISE THRESHOLD

Since some exercise is beneficial for relieving fatigue and boosting energy, you might think that more is better. But there is a tipping point, and you can actually end up doing too much of this good thing—and yet few people think about the risks of overexercising in the context of fatigue. The fact is, overexercising or overtraining occurs on a continuum, and the threshold for overexercising varies from one person to another, so it's important to tune in to how a particular exercise regimen makes *you* feel, rather than how it affects a friend, neighbor, or coworker.

One of the telltale signs of overexercising is fatigue. Other symptoms include persistent muscle soreness, an elevated resting heart rate, malaise, agitation or irritability, frequent illnesses or upper respiratory infections, insomnia or restless sleep, and loss of appetite. You might suspect you're suffering from overtraining if workouts that were once a breeze for you start feeling harder or if you experience a drop in performance (reduced speed or endurance, and the like).

At the far end of the continuum is overtraining syndrome (OTS), which can occur when people engage in excessive exercise without getting adequate rest. The combination of overdoing it without allowing sufficient time for rest and recovery can lead to harmful inflammation, neurological and hormonal changes, and undesirable effects on the central nervous system, including depressed mood, sleep disturbances, and bodywide fatigue, according to a 2012 review of the medical literature on OTS. Stress hormones (like cortisol) are produced in excess, and your body doesn't have time to repair itself. Excessive exercise can also place undue stress on your bones, joints, and muscles. Overtraining is a common phenomenon among professional and competitive athletes, but it happens to recreational exercisers, too.

Similarly, compulsive exercise disorder—which is like the exercise version of an eating disorder—can lead to physical symptoms of overtraining or psychological symptoms like severe anxiety (if you have to miss a workout, for instance) or a mental preoccupation with exercising. With this disorder, it's almost as if your exercise regimen comes to rule your life. I see this phenomenon in some of my hard-driving patients: They cruise from exercise class to exercise class on any given morning, or they head to the gym for a morning workout and fit in another one later in the day. Exercise becomes too much of a focal point for them, and many end up feeling drained, depleted, or dead tired and they can't understand why.

Sometimes these women take pride in being exercise junkies—but it's not healthy. Take my patient, Shannon, a mother of three in her early forties, who had recently reentered the workforce after being a stay-at-home mom when her kids were young. During the week, she was taking back-to-back Spinning classes at the crack of dawn and often one in the evening as well. After her morning workout, she did strength-training and isometric exercises with a trainer. Her diet was healthy—reasonable portions of nonprocessed foods such as meats, pasta, and veggies—but she felt she had to exercise that much to stay at her "ideal body weight," which was quite thin but not dangerously so.

When she came to see me last year, she complained of constant fatigue and low energy when she wasn't exercising, and she didn't have as much energy as she used to during her workouts. In addition to frequent dizziness, she was prone to occasional fainting spells when she first stood up in the morning. During the exam, I discovered that her resting heart rate was in the low 40s, occasionally dipping into the high 30s, most likely from her extreme fitness regimen. Her experience struck me as a clear example of how too much of a good thing (exercise) can be harmful in the end. The results of her blood work came back normal, so I referred her to a cardiologist, who confirmed that she had "athletic heart syndrome," a condition in which the heart becomes enlarged and the resting heart rate drops lower than normal as a result of intense exercise training; the cardiologist suggested she reduce her exercise regimen to prevent injury from fainting. Ironically, it wasn't until she sprained her ankle and was forced to take 2 months off that Shannon noted an increase in her energy. Once her ankle healed, however, she went right back to her usual regimen, which didn't do her energy any favors. The importance of tapering back on her exercise regimen is an ongoing discussion in each of our appointments, and I'm hoping that one day soon she'll turn the corner on that.

While heeding the maxims of "go hard or go home" or "giving your workout 110 percent" may sound like a surefire ticket to getting fit fast, the reality is that this approach can backfire, leading to increased exhaustion. If your workouts start leaving you more exhausted than energized, it may be time to dial down your routine and stop pushing yourself so long or so hard. Or you might need to take a break from exercise so your body and mind can recover, repair, and recharge. While you may worry about losing some of the fitness gains you've made, keep in mind that sometimes cutting back on the frequency, intensity, or duration of your workouts can actually help you get stronger because you'll be striking the right equilibrium between exercise and rest, the balance your body needs.

Where that balance lies is different for all of us. When I was in college, I spent a summer in Santa Cruz, California, which is a very health-conscious community. At the time, there were a lot of great vegetarian restaurants, free yoga and tai chi classes on the beach, and exercise enthusiasts everywhere. At most points during my ongoing battle with fatigue, I had forced myself to exercise at least a little bit (with light jogging, on the order of 2 miles three times per week), but the Santa Cruz summer seemed like the perfect place and time to amp up my fitness regimen. I hoped that building up my cardio-vascular endurance with more intense exercise would translate into more energy throughout the day.

So I increased my running to 4 to 6 miles four times a week and added some light weightlifting and aerobic exercise classes to my regimen. I was able to push through the exercise sessions, but I never felt as though my endurance was increasing over the 3-month period. What's more, I felt so tired afterward that I would need to take a nap, which perpetuated the frustrating feeling that I never had enough waking hours to accomplish what I wanted to. I experimented with morning versus afternoon workouts. I tried eating carbs and protein before and right after exercise. I tried everything I could think of to get more out of my workouts and reap more energy—but nothing seemed to help.

A few years later, I was diagnosed with chronic fatigue syndrome and learned that extreme exercise, which is essentially what I had been engaging in, exacerbates the condition. Now I have learned to strike the right balance for me: While getting no exercise worsens my fatigue, so does exercising too hard. Over time, I have discovered that power walking for 45 minutes to an hour, 5 days a week, seems to be the sweet spot that helps me stay fit and energized.

Now it's time for you to discover your own fitness formula, the one that relieves your fatigue; this will become an integral part of your personalized energy-boosting plan, as you'll see in Chapter 14. You may want to sample different forms of exercise and various venues to see what feels comfortable to you. If you've been sedentary until now, start by exercising at a low to moderate pace and gradually build up the length and intensity of your workouts as your body adjusts. Don't be afraid to tinker with the frequency, form, or duration of your workouts to see what feels right for your energy-boosting equation. Once you find the exercise sweet spot that works for you, make it a habit to go there regularly.

PART III

Sick and

Tired

CHAPTER SEVEN

Hormonal Havoc

WHEN IT COMES TO hormones, many women immediately think of reproductive hormones like estrogen and progesterone, the ones that fluctuate during the menstrual cycle, pregnancy, and the menopausal transition. These are certainly important, and they're an integral part of what makes us women. Among other things, estrogen enhances a woman's mood, memory, and overall sense of well-being and promotes deeper, more restorative sleep. When estrogen levels drop—during the second half of the menstrual cycle and during menopause—mood, energy, and motivation can suffer. Moreover, in the years leading up to menopause, women experience a drop in levels of testosterone (yes, it's mainly a male hormone, but women have it in lesser amounts, too) as the ovaries and adrenal glands slow the production of sex hormones; a drop in testosterone can lead to fatigue, decreased libido, and depression. So it's true that reproductive hormones affect how tired or energized you feel at various times in your life.

But sex-specific hormones are hardly the only ones that influence how we feel and function. The fact is, the endocrine system—a group of glands that produce and release various hormones—controls the body's metabolism, including its ability to convert nutrients into energy inside the cells, among many other functions. In addition to the thyroid, parathyroid, thymus, adrenal, and pituitary glands, the hypothalamus in the brain, the islet cells of the pancreas, the ovaries (in women), and the testes (in men) also produce hormones.

It helps to think of the hormonal (or endocrine) system as an elaborate cascade: Imagine one waterfall leading to another body of water, and that one leads to another waterfall, and so on, creating a beautiful system of waterways; a shift in one body of water can trigger a shift in the flow or volume of another. Hormones are similar in the sense that too much or too little of a particular hormone can affect the flow or balance of another hormone, potentially throwing multiple functions in your body out of whack. The challenge in diagnosing a hormonal imbalance is to identify a surplus or scarcity in one hormone before the rest of the body is affected.

Hormonal imbalances occur when one of the endocrine glands produces too much or too little of a particular hormone. Even the slightest imbalance may be considered an endocrine disorder, and these disorders cause fatigue, among other symptoms. Although various hormonal disorders have different ways of triggering fatigue, there are some commonalities. For one thing, many hormones play an important role in the energy cycle by regulating energy production and metabolism on a cellular level or by controlling the body's ability to convert nutrients into energy inside cells. Adrenal hormones like DHEA (short for dehydroepiandrosterone) and cortisol are released in a daily rhythm, and they work to maintain your energy, metabolize sugar by keeping insulin levels in the proper balance, support the immune system, and boost cognitive function in the brain; too little or too much DHEA or cortisol can set up a fatigue cascade. Meanwhile, stress causes increases in cortisol levels, which increases sugar in the bloodstream and insulin resistance; this wastes energy because it causes sugar, which should be burned as fuel, to end up being stored and ultimately converted into fat.

In addition, an excess of certain hormones is associated with chronic, low-level, systemic inflammation, which leads to fatigue. In a 2012 study, researchers from France compared fatigue levels among people with type 1 diabetes (an autoimmune condition) and type 2 diabetes (which involves chronic inflammation). They found that people with type 2 diabetes scored significantly higher on measures of fatigue, including general fatigue, physical fatigue, and reduced activity—and they had greater levels of inflammatory markers (including C-reactive protein, interleukin-6, and neopterin).

In terms of how inflammation causes fatigue, there are a few theories about the biological pathways that are involved. For starters, inflammation causes overstimulation of the immune system. It also may damage mitochondria, the energy sources within our cells that play a critical role in the production of adenosine triphosphate (ATP), which transports chemical energy within our cells. Because the cells don't have the necessary energy to function normally, cellular processes slow down, metabolism drops, and you experience fatigue. In addition, inflammation promotes oxidative stress, including the formation of cell-damaging free radicals. This causes fatigue by interfering with the mechanism that's responsible for delivering oxygen and nutrients to the cells; moreover, the cellular damage caused by free radicals may cause fatigue signals to be released in the brain. Some research suggests that inflammation decreases activity in the basal ganglia, the "reward center" in the brain that plays a critical role in motivation; the lower the activation, the less energy someone has.

For Women Only . . .

Polycystic ovary syndrome (PCOS, for short) is one of the most common endocrine/metabolic conditions in women. For reasons that aren't entirely understood, in women with PCOS, the ovaries make more androgens (male hormones) than normal, which affects the development and release of eggs during ovulation; the ovaries also often develop painless cysts. Excess insulin, which appears to increase production of androgens, also may be involved. Symptoms of PCOS include fatigue, irregular periods, excess body hair, thinning hair on the head, acne, weight gain, and depression. PCOS is linked with fertility problems as well. The disorder often clusters in families, so genetic factors likely play a role.

Not long ago, when I saw a 32-year-old friend at a mutual friend's birthday party, I noticed she had developed facial hair around her chin in a beardlike pattern. I decided to ask her what I hoped would be an inoffensive question, "How are you feeling?" She immediately told me she was exhausted and miserable. She said she couldn't lose weight despite "living on air and water"; she thought she might be going through early menopause because she had missed a few periods; and she had developed more prominent body hair that she regularly had removed with laser treatments. At my suggestion, she came by my office the next morning, and I tested her levels of DHEA (dehydroepiandrosterone) and testosterone. Sure enough, they were elevated, which confirmed she had PCOS.

Unfortunately, there isn't a cure for the disorder. Treatment usually addresses specific symptoms. Dietary changes—such as avoiding processed foods and foods with added sugar and sticking with whole grains, vegetables, fruits, and lean meats instead—can help with weight management and proper insulin function. In women who aren't trying to get pregnant, birth control pills can reduce male hormones, control the menstrual cycle, improve mood and energy, and help clear up acne. Spironolactone reduces male-pattern hair growth. In women who are trying to get pregnant, fertility medications may help.

Here's the important thing to remember: Women who have PCOS don't have to be at the mercy of this kind of hormonal imbalance; relief for bothersome symptoms can be obtained.

With many endocrine disorders, fatigue is one of the primary symptoms, but each of these disorders has a constellation of accompanying symptoms that are specific to it. That's why it's important to consider fatigue in the context of other symptoms, to help guide you to a possible diagnosis. Here's a look at how some of the most common endocrine disorders compare.

TYPE 2 DIABETES

During residency training, one of my fellow interns always had a 2-liter bottle of Evian in her white-coat pocket; it weighed down the jacket so much that one side hung a foot lower than the other. It became her signature look, and it was often joked about. She drank two to three bottles of water a day and had a stash of dozens in her call room. She never made it through a lecture without having to run off to pee. This woman, who was in her late twenties and slightly overweight but not obese, often complained of fatigue, but no one thought much of it because all medical residents are tired; that's just the way it is.

One day, she developed fever and extreme dizziness. When she went to the ER, her blood sugar was discovered to be more than 600 milligrams per deciliter (mg/dL)—dangerously high! She was diagnosed with type 2 diabetes and treated with an intravenous (IV) insulin drip for several days and then given oral medications to control her blood sugar. Gradually, her fatigue levels improved considerably.

Type 2 diabetes is the most common endocrine disorder in the United States. Approximately 30 million people in this country have some form of diabetes, and the vast majority have type 2. Type 2 diabetes occurs when the body does not produce enough insulin, a hormone that's needed to process and store sugar, or doesn't use insulin properly (a condition called insulin resistance). Your body needs insulin to be able to take the glucose (or sugar) it gets from the breakdown of food into the cells where it can be used for energy. When glucose builds up in the bloodstream instead of being transported into the body's cells, where it would be converted into energy, your cells become energy deprived. The result is that your body runs out of steam quickly even if you've had enough to eat; you also become dehydrated (as my fellow intern did), which results in fatigue. Over time, high blood sugar creates a variety of health problems—damaging your eyes, kidneys, nerves, or heart—but it also makes you feel tired and sluggish in the short term.

Indeed, when researchers at the University of Kansas Medical Center compared the presence and severity of fatigue among people with type 2 diabetes and people without the disease, they found that those with diabetes scored significantly higher on three different measures of fatigue than their healthy peers did. In another study, researchers at the University of Illinois at Chicago explored the relationship between fatigue and physiological, psychological, and lifestyle factors in women with type 2 diabetes: They found a significant link between fatigue and diabetes-related symptoms and emotional distress, depressive symptoms, a higher body mass index (BMI), and low levels of physical activity.

Insulin resistance is also a precursor to type 2 diabetes. With insulin resistance, your pancreas initially makes extra insulin to compensate for your body's poor use of the hormone, but gradually it can't keep up with the extra demand and produce enough insulin to keep your blood sugar at normal levels; this is when insulin resistance turns into full-blown diabetes. The risk is highest for people who are overweight, obese, or sedentary, or who have other family members with type 2 diabetes. In addition, type 2 diabetes is more common among certain ethnic groups, including African Americans, Latinos, Native Americans, Asian Americans, and Pacific Islanders.

One of the first signs of type 2 diabetes is dehydration, which causes symptoms like excessive thirst, increased urination, and fatigue. The fatigue is often accompanied by nausea, weakness, and shortness of breath. Other symptoms include slow-healing wounds, blurred vision, or unusual weight gain or weight loss. If you are experiencing these symptoms, you should see a doctor. It's easy to screen for type 2 diabetes with a fasting blood sugar test and a hemoglobin A1C test, which measures the average level of blood sugar over the previous 3 months. The earlier that type 2 diabetes is diagnosed and treated, the better it will be for your health and vitality.

If you are found to have diabetes, the choice of treatment depends in part on how high your blood sugar level is, your overall health, and what symptoms/complications you're experiencing. Some people with type 2 diabetes manage their condition—or even reverse it—with healthy dietary changes, exercise, and weight loss. Others require oral medications to bring their blood sugar levels into the target range. Different oral diabetes drugs have different mechanisms of action, but in general they work by upregulating the production and/or release of insulin by the pancreas. If the oral medications don't adequately control the diabetes, insulin injections may be required.

Another related condition that's often a precursor to type 2 diabetes and is associated with fatigue is metabolic syndrome (aka syndrome X), which is really a cluster of five risk factors for type 2 diabetes, heart disease, and stroke. These include elevated fasting blood sugar levels (100 mg/dL or

What's Weight Got to Do with It?

If you're overweight, you're at increased risk for a hormonal disorder that could drain your energy. Even if you don't have a disease such as type 2 diabetes or a thyroid disorder, if you're carrying extra pounds, you could have elevated estrogen levels. Here's why: Contrary to previous belief, fat cells aren't inert; they're metabolically active, and they produce the hormone estrogen, which can lead to excess levels of the female hormone in the body.

In the long run, this estrogen overload—or "estrogen dominance" in relation to progesterone levels—can raise a woman's risk of developing breast or uterine cancer. More immediately, it leads to a variety of unpleasant symptoms such as fatigue, depression, agitation, mood swings, memory loss, and further weight gain. While it's true that the falling estrogen levels that occur during menopause cause fatigue, too much estrogen can cause similar symptoms because the body's natural hormonal balance is upset. Plus, being overweight is tiring in its own right because carrying extra pounds places an undue burden on the body, one that drains your energy.

higher), excess abdominal fat (a waist circumference of 35 inches or more in women, 40 inches or more in men), high triglyceride levels (150 mg/dL or higher), low HDL (the "good") cholesterol levels (50 mg/dL or lower in women, 40 mg/dL or lower in men), and high blood pressure (130/85 or higher). If you have three of these five conditions, you are deemed to have metabolic syndrome, which means you have a higher likelihood of developing type 2 diabetes.

Lifestyle factors—including a nutritionally empty diet and sedentary habits—are the primary cause of metabolic syndrome. Fatigue is a common symptom of the syndrome. It comes from the condition itself (the excess weight, the elevated blood sugar, the cholesterol abnormalities, and/or the high blood pressure) as well as from the lifestyle factors that likely caused it. Generally, the treatment for metabolic syndrome involves an overhaul of your lifestyle habits—upgrading your diet, adding more physical activity, dropping excess weight, and quitting smoking—though sometimes medications are also used to treat certain components of the syndrome (like high blood pressure). The main goal is to reduce the risk of developing type 2 diabetes and cardiovascular disease, but a secondary one is to relieve symptoms that may accompany the condition.

THYROID DISORDERS

A small, butterfly-shaped gland at the base of the neck, the thyroid regulates the functioning of many organs in the body, including the heart, brain, liver, kidneys, bones, muscles, skin, and other organs. Thyroid hormones (T3 and T4) regulate energy and metabolism on a cellular level, in part by controlling the body's ability to convert nutrients into energy within cells. So if you have insufficient thyroid hormone, it means your energy factories can't use the food you've eaten to efficiently produce ATP, which transports chemical energy within cells, a scarcity that can make you feel tired. If your thyroid function is low (hypothyroidism), your metabolism, blood pressure, heart rate, digestion, and other functions can be slowed down, making you feel sluggish, lethargic, or as if you're in the midst of a full-blown energy crisis.

Hypothyroidism occurs most commonly in women over 60, but it affects younger women as well. It can happen after pregnancy or exposure to radiation (as a cancer treatment) or as a result of an autoimmune disorder (such as Hashimoto's disease). People with hypothyroidism often experience severe fatigue as their metabolism slows down, as well as weight gain, cold sensitivity, constipation, dry skin, joint or muscle pain, and depression.

Jennifer, a 45-year-old computer programmer who's married with two young children, had been suffering from progressive fatigue for 3 years when she came to see me. She reported taking frequent naps and feeling much too tired to do anything with her family when she got home from work. She was feeling depressed most of the time and more sensitive to criticism than ever before. For many years, maintaining a healthy weight had been effortless, but she suddenly found herself struggling to lose 25 pounds that she had gained in 2 years, even though she was sticking with the same healthy diet (primarily veggies and lean meats). In addition, she complained of dry skin and thinning hair. She thought she might be going through menopause, so she asked her ob-gyn to run tests, which were normal for her age. Jennifer came to see me because she "was sure something else was going on."

And indeed it was. On blood tests, her TSH level was elevated slightly, which meant she had borderline hypothyroidism. After being treated with levothyroxine (a synthetic thyroid hormone), her TSH level came into the normal range and her fatigue and other symptoms improved almost immediately. Within 6 months, she lost 10 pounds and regained enough energy to exercise three times a week.

On the other side of the spectrum is hyperthyroidism (an overactive thyroid). It may sound counterintuitive that a condition that revs you up could cause fatigue—after all, you might expect too much of this hormone to be energizing—but this happens in part because an overactive thyroid results in insomnia and other sleep disturbances. Plus, the stress the condition places on the body—thanks to a rapid pulse, elevated blood pressure, tremors, dizziness, mood swings, nervousness, diarrhea, increased sweating, shortness of breath, and other symptoms—can be draining.

If your thyroid function is in overdrive (as it is with hyperthyroidism), your thyroid gland makes too much thyroid hormone and your bodily processes are essentially sped up. Most cases of hyperthyroidism in women are caused by Graves' disease, which is an autoimmune disorder. Women are seven times more likely to get Graves' disease than men are, and it tends to run in families (smoking is also a risk factor). What's more, postpartum hyperthyroidism, which is called thyroiditis, affects 10 percent of women after they've given birth.

One of my patients, a 40-year-old media executive named Patricia, underwent a major cardiac procedure a year before our first visit. She complained of experiencing fatigue all day long—she had trouble waking up in the morning and falling asleep at night—and diarrhea, and she thought these symptoms might be related to the cardiac procedure. During the examination, she seemed nervous rather than tired, and she had a slight tremor in her hands and lower lip. Patricia also reported that she had been extremely emotional recently and that her boyfriend complained that she would burst into tears over minor disputes.

A blood test (to measure thyroid-stimulating hormone or TSH, T3, and T4) revealed that she had hyperthyroidism (specifically, Graves' disease, the most common form of hyperthyroidism in the United States), a condition her mother also had. I referred her to an endocrinologist, who administered radioactive iodine therapy to shrink the thyroid gland. After about 6 weeks, her symptoms, including her emotional reactivity and her fatigue, improved.

ADRENAL DISORDERS

One of the hottest disorders du jour, "adrenal fatigue" is a phrase used by some health-care practitioners to describe suboptimal adrenal gland function that's thought to be caused by emotional, mental, or physical stress. The theory behind adrenal fatigue is that if stress overwhelms your body, your adrenal glands cannot respond appropriately to the demand for stress hormones (like cortisol). This results in symptoms including waking up tired, chronic tiredness throughout the day, body aches, mental cloudiness, and an inability to focus or complete tasks. While adrenal fatigue is thought to cause severe, overwhelming fatigue in those who suffer from it, it is *not* a proven medical condition. Furthermore, lab tests for adrenal hormones (such as cortisol) tend to be normal with the condition, making diagnosis of the disorder even less clear.

While I'm not a complete naysayer about whether or not the condition is real, I would caution people against using any of the supplements that are promoted and sold under the guise of "adrenal health." Some of these actually contain extracts of human hormones, many of which are dangerous. For now, addressing and alleviating the triggers of so-called adrenal fatigue—namely, various forms of stress—is a better approach.

By contrast, adrenal insufficiency (aka Addison's disease) is a bona fide medical condition in which the adrenal glands produce too little of the hormone cortisol and often too little aldosterone, which helps maintain the body's balance of sodium and potassium to keep blood pressure normal. This hormonal insufficiency leads to muscle weakness and fatigue, weight loss and decreased appetite, hyperpigmentation (darkening of the skin), low blood pressure, salt cravings, low blood sugar, nausea or diarrhea, irritability, depression, loss of body hair, or sexual dysfunction.

Denise, a 40-something camera director at a local news station, had Hashimoto's thyroiditis that had been well controlled on Synthroid (levothyroxine; a synthetic thyroid hormone). Over the course of a year, she developed salt cravings, extreme fatigue, and dizziness upon standing, and she lost 20 pounds without trying. One day after the show, she fainted and was taken to the ER, where she was found to have dangerously low blood pressure, which responded to IV fluids, but it dropped again the moment the IV fluids were discontinued. Blood tests revealed that she had developed Addison's disease, which wasn't entirely surprising because patients with one autoimmune disease often develop another. Interestingly, once she was diagnosed, she realized that her skin had been more naturally "tan" recently, a key sign of the illness. Denise was treated with oral corticosteroids to replace the cortisol her adrenal glands weren't making; before long, her energy level rebounded.

Numerous other adrenal disorders are associated with fatigue. These include Cushing's disease, which is caused by a tumor or excessive growth of the pituitary gland, located at the base of the brain. In this condition, the pituitary gland releases too much adrenocorticotropic hormone (ACTH), which in turn stimulates the production and release of the stress hormone cortisol by the adrenal glands—an example of the hormonal cascade at work. Cushing's syndrome occurs when your body is exposed to high levels of the stress hormone cortisol for long periods of time, most commonly from chronic use of oral corticosteroid drugs. Besides fatigue, symptoms of both conditions include weight gain (especially around the midsection), stretch marks on the skin, easy bruising, slow wound healing, and headache. Both conditions are fairly rare and can be diagnosed with blood and urine tests to check ACTH and cortisol levels, respectively.

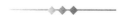

There's no question that hormonal disorders can be a serious drain on your energy and vitality. After all, your hormones affect nearly every part of your body, from head to toe, so when their levels are out of whack, you're unlikely to feel like your best self. Fortunately, there are numerous ways to calm just about every hormonal storm known to womankind and fix your fatigue in the process. The first step is to do a symptom inventory (which you'll find in Chapter 14) and then see your doctor to uncover the source of your fatigue and other symptoms. It may take a bit of time to figure out the right treatment for you, but with patience and perseverance, most women are able to find a way to repair their hormone-related energy drains.

CHAPTER EIGHT

Under Friendly Fire: Autoimmune Diseases

INSIDE YOUR BODY IS an amazing defense department. It consists of a complex and intricate network of specialized cells, proteins, tissues, and organs, and it is designed to protect you from foreign invaders, including bacteria, viruses, fungi, parasites, and toxins. It's called the immune system, and it works around the clock to help you stay healthy, fight illnesses, prevent diseases, and heal from wounds, infections, and injuries. When the immune system works well, the results are brilliant; when it doesn't, well, not so much.

The immune system has a variety of responsibilities, many of which fall under two different forms of protection: natural immunity and acquired immunity. Natural immunity is created by the body's natural barriers, such as the skin and the protective substances (such as mucus) in the mouth, urinary tract, and surface of the eye. Natural immunity also occurs when a mother passes antibodies on to her baby during pregnancy. Acquired immunity, by contrast, develops as you're exposed to specific germs, toxins, and infectious microorganisms. The immune system starts to "remember" these foreign particles (antigens) and produces specific antibodies (specialized proteins that block specific antigens) to them. When a foreign particle enters the body again, the immune system releases antibodies to attack it and prevent that illness from recurring (as in the case of chicken pox).

To function at an optimal level, the immune system needs to be able to distinguish between the cells, tissues, and organs that belong to you and the germs and other foreign invaders that don't. When that ability becomes flawed, when your body begins having trouble telling the difference between what's *you* and what's *foreign*, it makes autoantibodies that attack normal cells by mistake. Meanwhile, regulatory T cells, which normally keep the immune system in check, fail to maintain "self-tolerance" and suppress immune reactions to the body's own normal cells or to harmless substances (such as allergens). This leads to an erroneous or misguided attack on your own healthy cells, causing the damage that's associated with autoimmune diseases.

Approximately 50 million people in the United States—the vast majority of them women, especially women of childbearing age—suffer from autoimmune ailments. There are more than 80 known types of autoimmune diseases, and different types affect different body parts, although they universally cause fatigue and general malaise. Outside of that, they can cause just about any physical symptom that exists from head to toe, including chest pain, joint pain, digestive distress, fever, and vision changes. Moreover, autoimmune issues affect every organ system, and many women suffer from more than one autoimmune disease at a given time. The autoimmune disorders that are most closely associated with fatigue include lupus, rheumatoid arthritis, multiple sclerosis, primary biliary cirrhosis, myasthenia gravis, and Sjögren's syndrome.

One classic sign of these autoimmune disorders is inflammation, which manifests as redness, heat, pain, and/or swelling, depending on what part of the body is affected. If the disease affects the joints, as in rheumatoid arthritis, it causes joint pain and stiffness and loss of function. If inflammation attacks the skin, as it does in scleroderma, vitiligo, and lupus, it causes rashes, blisters, and color changes to the skin. But inflammation may be invisible to the naked eye if it's occurring internally. For example, if it affects the thyroid, as in Graves' disease and thyroiditis, it causes tiredness, weight gain, and muscle aches.

But no matter how it's manifested, inflammation ultimately causes fatigue through a number of biological pathways. These include overstimulation of the immune system, damage to mitochondria (the energy sources within our cells), and the promotion of oxidative stress including the formation of cell-damaging free radicals (which can interfere with the mechanism responsible for delivering oxygen and nutrients to the cells). Inflammation can also trigger the stress response system in the brain (the hypothalamic-pituitary-adrenal axis, or HPA axis), and, over time, the chronic effects of stress hormones like cortisol deplete a person's energy. In addition, autoimmune diseases like rheumatoid arthritis and lupus often cause muscle and joint pain that makes it difficult for sufferers to get a good night's sleep, which naturally contributes to their exhaustion.

Autoimmune diseases affect women three times more often than they do men. No one knows exactly why this is, but there are three primary theories. One has to do with X chromosomes: Men have a pair of XY chromosomes while women have a pair of XX chromosomes. Most genes on women's second X chromosome are silent, but a few that play a role in immune function are expressed, which means that women have more active genes that are involved in immunity than men do. We don't know exactly why this is. But the theory is that this extra activity could lead to immune function gone awry, making women more susceptible to autoimmune diseases.

Another theory involves hormones: Testosterone (which men have more of) generally suppresses the body's response to infection, while estrogen (which women have more of) boosts it; the idea is that since women have a more vigorous immune response in general, their immune systems are more likely to become overactive and turn against a woman's own cells, leading to autoimmune diseases. Yet another hypothesis has to do with the presence of someone else's cells in your body (namely, during pregnancy): During pregnancy and childbirth, there's a significant exchange of cells between mother and child. The cells that don't naturally belong to each person are usually cleared by both people within weeks after childbirth. The thinking is that in some people, the cells are not entirely cleared and they stay in the host permanently, triggering the immune system to recognize the body's own healthy cells as foreign and attack them.

While the exact cause of autoimmune diseases is unknown, studies have shown that triggers can include exposure to bacteria and viruses, certain medications, and chemical and environmental exposures. The immune system has an elaborate system of checks and balances to prevent the destruction of the body's own tissues—but some data suggest that a strong or chronic immune response to infections (bacterial, viral, and parasitic ones) disrupts this balance and leads to autoimmune diseases. No single infection has been found to be responsible, and many different infections may be connected to any given autoimmune disorder. Of course, not everyone who gets these infections will develop an autoimmune disorder, which suggests the trigger may be partly genetic or may involve other environmental factors, too. Still, some patterns have emerged, linking certain autoimmune disorders with specific infectious viruses and bacterial infections (at this point, these are theoretical links, not established causes and effects). Here's a look:

♦ **Multiple sclerosis:** Epstein–Barr virus and measles virus

♦ **Type 1 diabetes:** Coxsackievirus B4, cytomegalovirus, mumps virus, and rubella virus

♦ **Rheumatoid arthritis:** Epstein–Barr virus, hepatitis C virus, *Escherichia coli* bacteria, and mycobacteria

♦ **Lupus:** Epstein–Barr virus

♦ **Myocarditis:** Coxsackievirus B3, cytomegalovirus, and chlamydia (a bacterial infection)

♦ **Myasthenia gravis:** Hepatitis C virus and herpes simplex virus types 1 and 2

♦ **Guillain–Barré syndrome:** Epstein–Barr virus, cytomegalovirus, and campylobacter bacteria

Theories aside, it's well established that autoimmune diseases tend to cluster in families. But in most cases, a specific genetic link has not been pinpointed. Some autoimmune diseases have a greater effect on people of certain racial backgrounds than others: For example, type 1 diabetes is more common among Caucasians, while lupus tends to be most severe among African American and Hispanic people. One of the greatest hallmarks of autoimmune diseases is that they are notoriously hard to diagnose. This is partly because their symptoms can wax and wane, fluctuating between flare-ups (worsening of symptoms) and remissions (periods of no symptoms). It's also because no single test can confirm or deny the presence of a particular autoimmune disease.

What follows is a high-altitude view of the most common autoimmune diseases that affect women in the United States. Almost all are heralded by the top symptom of fatigue. There are dozens of others, including skin conditions like scleroderma and vitiligo, nerve and muscle conditions like myasthenia gravis, and digestive disorders like celiac disease and inflammatory bowel disease (which you will read about in Chapter 10)—but to explore them all would take five books. So I am sticking with the primary suspects here. If you see your own experience in the symptom profiles that follow, my hope is that you'll make an appointment to see your doctor—pronto!—so you can get the proper diagnosis and treatment sooner, not later.

SYSTEMIC LUPUS ERYTHEMATOSUS

A disease that causes inflammation that can damage the joints, skin, heart, lungs, kidneys, and other parts of the body, systemic lupus erythematosus (aka SLE or just "lupus") affects an estimated 1.5 million people in the United States, the vast majority of them women. The age of onset is typically between 15 and 44. Symptoms include fever, fatigue, weight loss, hair loss, mouth sores, a telltale butterfly-shaped rash across the nose and cheeks, muscle pain, painful or swollen joints, chest pain, shortness of breath, headaches, and dizziness. No two cases of lupus are exactly alike, but nearly all of them feature fatigue and fever—and are marked by flares and remissions. Sometimes the illness is hard to pin down because there are times when the person feels fine.

A friend of a friend, Cindy is a model-actress in her late thirties who lives with her boyfriend and their 2-year-old daughter in New York City. After the baby's birth, she started suffering from extreme fatigue, anxiety, and heart palpitations. At her two postpartum visits, her thyroid antibodies were tested, and they were within the normal range. Two years later, she was still complaining of crippling fatigue; some days, she couldn't get out of bed, so she would just read and watch TV with her daughter. She hadn't been able to go back to work. To make matters worse, her health insurance had expired. Her friends and family members were worried about her because they thought she was overwhelmed and possibly depressed.

One day, our mutual friend called me to ask about symptoms of blood clots because her friend had developed sudden swelling and pain in her ankles and knees. I had her come to the office and immediately noticed that her usually flawless skin had what looked like rosacea or severe acne across the bridge of her nose and cheeks. Because I suspected she might have lupus, I drew her blood to test for antinuclear antibodies (ANA), the presence of which indicates an overstimulated immune system. The result of her ANA test was highly positive, and a later test confirmed she had lupus-specific antigens. She told me that her mother had died relatively young of a sudden cardiac problem that was never clarified; I suspect it might have been lupus-related carditis (inflammation of the heart). Shortly after Cindy started taking Plaquenil (hydroxychloroquine; a disease-modifying antirheumatic drug, or DMARD), which reduces pain and swelling, along with other medications, she experienced an improvement in her symptoms, including relief from her previously relentless fatigue.

While no single test can diagnose lupus, a combination of blood tests for specific markers—such as ANA and anti-double-stranded DNA (anti-dsDNA), anti-Smith, and antiphospholipid antibodies, as well as C3, C4, or

CH50 complement levels—plus a physical examination (including taking a medical history of signs and symptoms) confirms the presence of the autoimmune disease. In some cases, imaging studies of the heart, lungs, and kidneys are done to look for damage.

Nonsteroidal anti-inflammatory drugs (NSAIDs, like ibuprofen and naproxen) are often used as a first-line treatment for the mild pain, inflammation, and fever that occur in the early stages of lupus. Once the disease begins to progress, antimalarial drugs like Plaquenil are considered. These have revolutionized treatment: They help slow the disease's course and minimize symptoms for many women. In severe forms of lupus, corticosteroid drugs (like prednisone) and other immunosuppressant medications play an important role, but because of their side effects profile, they are generally reserved for use after other options have failed. Some people with lupus also require other types of drugs to treat conditions that often go hand in hand with lupus—such as diuretics (for fluid retention), antihypertensive drugs (for high blood pressure), and antibiotics (for infections).

RHEUMATOID ARTHRITIS

Nearly 1.5 million people in the United States have rheumatoid arthritis (RA). The autoimmune disease is three times more common among women, with the onset usually occurring between the ages of 30 and 60. RA happens when the immune system mistakenly attacks the joints—especially the lining of the joints (the synovial membrane)—throughout the body, which leads to erosion of the cartilage and bone and sometimes to deformed joints. It can also affect the skin, eyes, lungs, and blood vessels.

The most common symptoms of RA include fatigue, joint pain, and tender, warm, swollen joints. Fever and weight loss are subtle, early signs of the disease. Morning joint stiffness that lasts a few hours is common, too, and often you can see inflammation of the small joints in the hands and wrists.

No single test can confirm or deny the presence of RA. The autoimmune disease is usually diagnosed by a combination of physical examination and blood tests to measure the erythrocyte sedimentation rate and C-reactive protein (both are markers of inflammation), rheumatoid factor (an antibody found in the majority of people with RA), and anti-cyclic citrullinated peptide antibodies (another marker for the diagnosis and prognosis of RA). Since RA can cause erosions at the ends of the bones within a joint, sometimes an x-ray, ultrasound, or MRI (magnetic resonance imaging) scan is done to look for erosions. The absence of erosions doesn't rule out RA, though; it could just mean it's in an early stage and hasn't led to noticeable damage to your bones.

There's no cure for RA, but there are medications that ease symptoms, reduce inflammation, and slow the progression of the disease. NSAIDs (such as ibuprofen and naproxen) are the first-line treatment for mild pain, swelling, and fever in the disease's early stages. Corticosteroids (like prednisone) reduce swelling and pain, but they cause significant side effects (such as elevated blood sugar and thinning bones) when they're used for long periods. DMARDs (such as methotrexate and Plaquenil) were once reserved for severe, chronic RA, but they are now started early on in the disease to try to spare joints and tissues from permanent damage. Biologic agents such as tumor necrosis factor alpha inhibitors and immunosuppressant drugs (such as cyclosporine) are also commonly used.

There isn't a single drug that works for everyone with RA. But with some experimentation—and a dose of patience—many people find treatments that are very effective. The goal of treatment is to achieve a state of remission (when inflammation and other symptoms are very low or nonexistent). As your physician monitors your symptoms, your disease activity, and the effects of your medications, he or she may add or switch your medications periodically or adjust the dosage. Good self-care is also an integral part of the equation: Staying physically active maintains flexibility and keeps the muscles strong, which in turn protects your joints. Managing your weight,

Flicking the Cellular Switch?

At this point, there's no cure for autoimmune diseases—but there is hope on the horizon. In a study published in September 2014, researchers at the University of Bristol in the United Kingdom reported that they may have discovered a way to "turn off" autoimmune diseases such as multiple sclerosis, lupus, and type 1 diabetes at the cellular level. The scientists were able to selectively target the cells that cause autoimmune disease and turn off their aggression against the body's own tissues while converting those cells into ones that could protect against disease. This approach involves using fragments of the proteins the immune cells would normally attack and "teaching" the cells to identify the proteins as harmless.

This type of conversion has been used with allergies, but its application to autoimmune diseases is quite recent. The process is called immunotherapy, and if it works in this context, it could be a major breakthrough for people with autoimmune diseases. It would provide a highly targeted approach to halting autoimmune diseases without the side effects of the drugs that are currently used and without affecting healthy cells.

consuming a nutritious diet, and getting adequate rest on a daily basis are important measures, too.

SJÖGREN'S SYNDROME

You may not have heard of Sjögren's syndrome, but more than four million people in the United States have it—and 90 percent of them are women. This is a disease in which the immune system's white blood cells attack the mucous membranes and the glands that produce moisture in the body (such as tears and saliva). Sjögren's syndrome also causes problems with the kidneys, lungs, liver, pancreas, blood vessels, gastrointestinal system, and central nervous system. People who have it also may experience severe fatigue and joint swelling or pain.

Symptoms vary from one person to another but often include dryness of the mouth, eyes, nose, or vagina as well as trouble swallowing, a loss of taste or smell, an increase in dental cavities and decay, a hoarse voice, and swollen salivary glands. Because symptoms of Sjögren's are similar to those of other autoimmune diseases (including lupus, rheumatoid arthritis, and multiple sclerosis) or other health conditions (such as fibromyalgia or chronic fatigue syndrome), it takes an average of 4.7 years for someone to get an accurate diagnosis after the onset of symptoms. Complicating matters, in about 50 percent of people with Sjögren's, the disease occurs by itself—but in the other 50 percent, it occurs along with other autoimmune diseases such as rheumatoid arthritis or lupus.

There isn't a single test to diagnose Sjögren's definitively. So physicians often rely on a battery of blood tests (including a complete blood count, ANA, and specific Sjögren's-associated SS-A and SS-B antibodies) as well as other blood tests to rule out other autoimmune conditions. Additional tests may include an eye moisture exam (called a Schirmer's test) and salivary gland function tests or a salivary gland biopsy.

Once Sjögren's is diagnosed, treatment involves addressing specific symptoms, such as using moisturizing drops for dry eyes and dry mouth. In more severe forms of the disease, oral drugs such as NSAIDs, DMARDs (like Plaquenil), and immunosuppressive drugs may be prescribed to treat internal manifestations of the autoimmune disease. Treatment is highly individualized and really depends on a woman's symptoms and the manifestations of Sjögren's.

Melanie, a 47-year-old former marketing executive turned stay-at-home mom, was diagnosed with depression and treated with antidepressants and psychotherapy following the birth of her youngest son, now 3. She was complaining of constant fatigue and dry mouth, which she attributed to side effects of the antidepressants—but changing drugs several times didn't help. It wasn't long before her eyes started to bother her. Her ophthalmologist diagnosed her with dry eye syndrome, but rather than simply prescribing moisturizing eye drops, he went the extra mile and gave Melanie blood tests. Sure enough, Sjögren's syndrome was confirmed by the presence of specific antibodies. Melanie was given salivary-gland stimulators to help with the dry mouth symptoms. She didn't want to take systemic medications, so she has chosen to live with her waxing and waning symptoms of fatigue and occasional joint pain.

MULTIPLE SCLEROSIS

A disease in which the immune system attacks the protective coating (the myelin) around nerve fibers in the central nervous system, multiple sclerosis (MS) affects an estimated 400,000 people in the United States. It is two to three times more common among women than men and usually strikes between the ages of 20 and 50. While the cause of MS isn't known, genetic factors likely play a role in susceptibility, and environmental triggers (including living farther from the equator, smoking, and certain viruses) may be involved, too.

Because it affects the central nervous system, MS damages the brain and spinal cord, leading to a wide array of symptoms including muscle weakness, blurred or double vision, tremors, numbness and tingling in the extremities, dizziness and vertigo, and trouble with coordination and balance. This is because the central nervous system comprises nerves that carry messages between the body and the brain, and these messages control muscle movements that are involved in walking and talking, among other activities.

Fatigue occurs in about 80 percent of people who have MS. For some MS sufferers, fatigue is also the presenting symptom—it's the one that comes before other MS signs become apparent. Even though many people with

MS wake up feeling tired, MS-related fatigue tends to get worse as the day goes on; it's also exacerbated by heat and humidity.

Since there isn't a single test for MS, the autoimmune disease can be difficult to diagnose. In fact, the diagnosis is often missed, delayed, or even misdiagnosed as something else. This is partly because the symptoms, course, and severity of the disease vary considerably from person to person. To make the diagnosis, a physician must find evidence of damage in at least two separate areas of the central nervous system *and* evidence that the damage occurred at least a month apart *and* rule out all other possible diagnoses. Diagnosis is made on the basis of a careful medical history, a thorough neurologic examination, and various tests such as an MRI scan to detect areas of myelin that have been damaged by MS.

Treatment generally involves medications that are used to modify the course of MS, treat relapses (or attacks), and manage symptoms. A variety of disease-modifying agents are available, and more are in the developmental pipeline; relapses are often treated with corticosteroids. Meanwhile, a host of different medications are used to manage specific symptoms of MS, from bladder dysfunction, dizziness, and spasticity to pain and fatigue.

PERNICIOUS ANEMIA

An autoimmune disorder in which the body does not have enough healthy red blood cells or hemoglobin, pernicious anemia is caused by an impaired uptake of vitamin B_{12} from the diet. With this condition, the immune system mistakenly attacks cells that secrete intrinsic factor, a protein made in the stomach. Your intestines need intrinsic factor to absorb vitamin B_{12} from your diet; without enough intrinsic factor, the condition results in a severe B_{12} deficiency. This is a problem because vitamin B_{12} is needed to make healthy red blood cells and to keep the nervous system working properly.

The most common symptom of pernicious anemia is tiredness. When you don't have enough healthy red blood cells, you feel weak and may experience shortness of breath, as well as tingling or numbness in the hands and feet. Severe or long-lasting pernicious anemia damages the heart, brain, nerves, and bones and can cause memory loss and problems in the digestive tract. Pernicious anemia is picked up by routine blood tests (such as a complete blood count) along with more specific markers such as high levels of homocysteine and methylmalonic acid. The presence of intrinsic factor antibodies can clinch the diagnosis.

Fortunately, treatment of pernicious anemia is pretty simple: monthly vitamin B_{12} injections (or a newer nasal spray or gel) for life. This is what one of my patients, Grace, a 50-year-old TV producer, discovered a few years ago. After having gastric bypass surgery, she had lost 130 pounds over the course of 4 years and was relishing her newfound abundance of energy, enjoyment of exercise, and general vitality. I remember her telling me that she'd never felt better, not even as a child.

Then she suddenly hit a roadblock: Over a 6-month period, she developed shortness of breath and debilitating fatigue. It got to the point where she found it difficult to sit at her desk and work without feeling an intense need to take a nap. She also complained about tingling and coldness in her hands and feet. A blood test revealed anemia from a B_{12} deficiency, a common side effect of gastric bypass surgery because the part of the stomach that releases intrinsic factor has been removed. Once Grace began getting monthly B_{12} injections, her get-up-and-go returned.

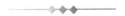

So now you know that autoimmune diseases strike women disproportionately—and they can seriously compromise your vim and vigor, state of health, and quality of life. That's why if you're in the midst of a personal energy crisis, it's wise to tune in to other symptoms that suggest your body has launched an internal mutiny. If your immune system is attacking healthy cells, tissues, and organs by mistake, you'll want to take steps to halt those effects before permanent damage occurs. To that end, you and your physician will want to work closely to devise a plan to manage your symptoms, minimize or prevent flare-ups, and slow the progression of the autoimmune disease. Right now, there isn't a cure for most autoimmune diseases, but researchers are making progress in looking for new ways to treat them, reduce long-term complications, and improve the quality of life for those who have them. In addition to taking medications, there's a lot you can do to feel better—namely, by adopting the lifestyle changes that are described in Chapter 14. By sticking with a healthy diet, regular physical activity, good stress management strategies, and effective sleep hygiene techniques, you will begin to reclaim your vitality as you search for the right treatment for you.

CHAPTER NINE

Organs in Distress

MY FRIEND JULIE, A 37-year-old fashion executive, used to be a serious athlete—she played Division I basketball and lacrosse in college—and still works out 5 days a week. One day at nursery school drop-off, she commented that she must be getting old because she's completely exhausted after walking her daughter to school and gets winded after every Spinning and core fusion class she takes. When I asked for details, she said that for the last couple of months, she hadn't been able to catch her breath for the latter half of her exercise classes, and afterward, she felt so tired that she'd need to nap. Even several hours after exercising, she still felt wiped out.

It didn't sound like a heart problem because she wasn't experiencing chest pain or pressure, pain down the arms or in the neck or jaw, or heart palpitations—the classic symptoms of heart disease. Plus, Julie is slim and fit and has no history of high blood pressure or cholesterol abnormalities. Still, I sent her for a stress echocardiogram, which immediately showed myocardial ischemia, which means that an area of her heart wasn't getting enough oxygen. Julie went straight to the hospital for an emergency angioplasty because she was at high risk for having a heart attack: A major coronary artery had a 90 percent blockage, while her other arteries were clear. Once the artery was surgically opened, a stent was put in to keep it that way, and Julie made a full recovery.

We don't mean to, but many of us take our organs for granted, which isn't surprising since a healthy heart, lungs, kidneys, and liver generally function automatically. We don't have to do anything special to make them run efficiently. They simply do their respective jobs—pumping blood throughout the body, breathing in oxygen from the air and breathing out carbon dioxide, preventing the buildup of wastes and excess fluid, removing toxins from the blood and metabolizing drugs, among other tasks. All of this happens without our conscious awareness—that is, until something goes wrong, as it did in Julie's case.

The truth is, diseases and disorders involving the heart, lungs, kidneys, and liver are more common than you might think—and fatigue is one of the primary complaints with these conditions. Each one will have its own set of accompanying symptoms (such as shortness of breath in the case of heart and lung diseases or back pain in the case of kidney disorders), and different forms of organ dysfunction cause fatigue in different ways. With heart problems, for example, people typically feel tired because the heart's pumping ability is decreased, causing less than the optimal amount of blood to reach the muscles and tissues of the body; fatigue also occurs because waste products aren't being removed as quickly or efficiently as they should be. By contrast, lung diseases contribute to ongoing fatigue by causing low oxygen levels or elevated carbon dioxide levels in the body, by making the work of breathing more laborious, or by making the person susceptible to frequent respiratory infections, which can cause fatigue by triggering the release of immune cells called cytokines. Meanwhile, with kidney or liver dysfunction, fatigue stems from the buildup of waste products or toxins in the blood, from electrolyte or fluid imbalances, or from inflammation.

Whatever the underlying mechanism might be, this much is clear: Each form of organ dysfunction creates a slow, insidious energy drain from the entire system (namely, the body). This is why any woman who has significant, persistent fatigue should be checked for cardiac (heart) and pulmonary (lung) disease as well as kidney and liver problems. Sometimes, too, dysfunction with one organ is linked to problems with another. This is true of heart disease and kidney problems; some lung conditions; and nonalcoholic fatty liver disease and chronic kidney disease, for instance. Because of this, it's important to catch these disorders as early as possible to prevent a detrimental domino effect among the organ systems.

What follows is a bird's-eye view of the most common forms of organ dysfunction that drain your energy. There are many others, but I address the primary suspects here. If you recognize your own experience in the symptom profiles that follow, I urge you to make an appointment to see your doctor as soon as possible.

HEART PROBLEMS

Believe it or not, heart disease—not breast cancer or any other form of cancer—is the leading killer of US women, causing one in three deaths each year (that amounts to nearly a woman every minute!), according to the American Heart Association. Approximately 6.6 million women in the United States currently have heart disease, and yet only one out of every five women in this country believes that heart disease is the greatest threat to her health. That's a shame, because there's so much we can all do to reduce our risk (including following the lifestyle modifications that are recommended in this book).

For women, fatigue is frequently one of the first symptoms of heart disease (aka cardiovascular disease). This may seem surprising, since many people associate chest pain with the condition, but it makes physiological sense if you think about it this way: Cardiovascular disease is caused by narrowed, blocked, or stiffened blood vessels that prevent your heart, brain, or other parts of your body from receiving enough blood, and this is what leads to a heart attack or stroke. But before that cardiac event happens, it's the diminished bloodflow to vital areas of the body that makes you feel tired. In a 2003 study of 515 female heart attack survivors, researchers at the University of Arkansas found that 70 percent of the women reported unusual fatigue in the weeks before the cardiac event, whereas only 30 percent had chest discomfort (a classic symptom in men) during that same period. What's more, fatigue was a symptom in women with dangerously clogged arteries that escaped notice on heart scans, according to a report from the Women's Ischemia Syndrome Evaluation (WISE) study.

When people have heart failure, the body diverts blood away from the less vital areas (such as the muscles in the arms and legs) so that it can send blood to the heart, brain, and kidneys—another pattern that leads to sluggishness and fatigue. People with heart failure may feel tired all the time and have difficulty performing daily activities such as walking, climbing stairs, or carrying groceries. Other heart-related conditions also cause fatigue. These include:

♦ **Cardiac arrhythmias:** A heart arrhythmia is basically an abnormal heart rhythm that can be caused by hyperthyroidism, electrolyte disturbances, or undiagnosed heart valve damage (which can happen from narrowing, leaking, or improper closing of the valves). With arrhythmias, the heart may beat too quickly, too slowly, or simply irregularly. In addition to fatigue, symptoms include a fluttering sensation in your chest, a racing heartbeat (tachycardia), a slow heartbeat (bradycardia), chest pain or discomfort, shortness of breath, light-headedness, dizziness, fainting, or almost fainting.

♦ **Congenital heart defects:** Unfortunately, subtler or less serious congenital heart defects (ones you're born with) often aren't diagnosed until late childhood or even adulthood. Signs and symptoms include getting short of breath easily during exercise or other forms of physical activity, tiring easily during exercise or physical activity, and having recurring bouts of swelling in the hands, ankles, or feet.

- **Cardiomyopathy:** A group of diseases affecting the heart muscle, cardiomyopathy involves a thickening and stiffening of the heart muscle, or a stretching and weakening of the heart muscle, either of which makes the heart unable to pump blood effectively. Cardiomyopathy may stem from genetic or congenital causes, or it can be caused by damage from infections or autoimmune diseases (such as lupus). Besides fatigue, symptoms include swelling of the legs, ankles, and feet; breathlessness with exertion or even at rest; irregular heartbeats that feel rapid, pounding, or fluttering; dizziness, light-headedness, and fainting.

Four years ago, one of my patients called me about her daughter Ella, a 22-year-old college student who had been complaining of severe fatigue for 4 months. Ella had recently quit the basketball team because she found the training too rigorous. She was spending most of each day in bed studying, and she thought she may have had mono because it was going around her dorm. During their last visit, her mother noticed that Ella seemed easily winded with exertion or movement, but her daughter said she was just tired. The campus doctors had diagnosed her with a "viral syndrome," characterized by lingering fatigue after the infection. I suggested to her mom that Ella come see me when she was home for break.

Two days before her appointment, Ella lost consciousness while walking the dog, and she was rushed to the hospital. She was diagnosed with dilated cardiomyopathy—it turns out she likely had a genetic propensity toward it since her maternal grandmother and one aunt died suddenly at young ages of unclear cardiac causes. Ella was treated with ACE inhibitors to increase the pumping strength of her heart, and she had a pacemaker put in. Her fatigue symptoms have improved, but with this condition Ella will require long-term treatment.

- **Cardiac infections:** There are three major types of heart infections—pericarditis, which affects the tissue surrounding the heart (the pericardium); myocarditis, which affects the muscular middle layer of the walls of

Medication Malaise?

When it comes to exhaustion that's related to organ dysfunction, there's an added challenge for people with heart disease: Many of the medications that are used to treat heart disease cause or exacerbate fatigue. Some examples:

♦ **BETA-BLOCKERS** slow down the pumping action of the heart and depress parts of the central nervous system—both of these effects can lead to fatigue.

♦ **DIURETICS**, which are often used to treat high blood pressure, can deplete the body of minerals and electrolytes like potassium and sodium; this may leave you feeling drained, weak, and achy.

♦ **STATINS**, used to treat cholesterol abnormalities, may interfere with the production of energy at the cellular level and halt the production of satellite cells in the muscles, which can lead to muscle weakness and pain.

If you experience a worsening of your fatigue while taking any of these medications, your best bet is to talk to your doctor about whether you can switch to a different drug or another approach to treat your blood pressure or cholesterol abnormalities.

the heart (the myocardium); and endocarditis, which affects the inner membrane that separates the chambers and valves of the heart (the endocardium). Symptoms vary slightly with each type of infection but may include fever, shortness of breath, weakness or fatigue, swelling in the legs or abdomen, changes in heart rhythms, a dry or persistent cough, or unusual skin rashes or spots.

LUNG DISEASES

Lung diseases are among the most common medical conditions in the world, and the number of women in the United States who are being diagnosed with lung disease is on the rise. The three most common types in women are asthma, chronic obstructive pulmonary disease (COPD), and lung cancer, which is the leading killer cancer among women and men alike. Almost all lung diseases cause fatigue as a primary symptom. In fact, fatigue is three times more common among people suffering from lung disease than in healthy adults. When COPD patients are asked to name the symptoms that worsen their quality of life, fatigue ranks almost as high as shortness of breath.

When Mackenzie, a 28-year-old graduate student in art history, came to see me, she immediately asked for a test for anemia. She had felt tired for several years and described waking up feeling unrested and having her fatigue worsen as the day progressed; she also coughed at night, which compromised the quality of her sleep. Mackenzie had started relying on energy drinks to help her stay alert and focused for studying. She would jog 2 or 3 days a week and noticed she felt more tired the day after exercising.

The cause was mysterious because she didn't have any shortness of breath or chest pain, and the results of her blood tests came back normal. But when I examined her, I noticed a faint wheeze when she'd exhale, so I referred her for spirometry and bronchoprovocation testing, which measure lung function. These revealed that she had cough-variant asthma, a form of asthma that causes coughing rather than wheezing as its main symptom. In Mackenzie's case, it was triggered especially by exercise and cold air, but her symptoms and fatigue persisted long past her exercise sessions. Treating her asthma with a bronchodilator resolved her symptoms, including her fatigue.

There are a number of different mechanisms through which lung diseases cause fatigue, depending largely on how a specific disease affects the lungs. With COPD, people may experience low oxygen levels or elevated carbon dioxide levels, both of which are sedating and can compromise thinking abilities. Most asthma sufferers are able to maintain normal oxygen levels, but the work of breathing is more difficult, which contributes to fatigue. Meanwhile, people who have any form of lung disease often suffer from frequent respiratory infections that can trigger the release of cytokines. These are small proteins that act as mediators between cells. They prime the immune response but also make you feel tired. (The evolutionary theory regarding cytokine-mediated fatigue is that the release of these proteins makes you slow down and rest, thereby conserving the body's resources for fighting an infection.) Last, people with chronic lung diseases typically end up spending less time outdoors and more time being sedentary in an effort to avoid exacerbating their shortness of breath. This pattern leads to a reduction in exercise tolerance, decreased strength and endurance, and a never-ending cycle of inactivity causing fatigue and fatigue causing inactivity.

When Elaine, a 65-year-old widow with emphysema, came to see me, she complained that she felt like a "100-year-old woman." Although she had never smoked, she lived and worked at home with her late husband, who had smoked two to three packs a day (he passed away from lung cancer 5 years before our visit). Elaine developed emphysema (a chronic lung disease that causes difficulty with exhaling) from exposure to secondhand smoke. Her condition was well controlled with bronchodilators, she didn't complain of shortness of breath, and her blood oxygen levels were normal on a pulse oximeter exam in my office. She said she tried "never to move" so that she wouldn't trigger a bout of coughing, and she said she had so little energy that getting to and from the bathroom was becoming a challenge.

Our visit was one of the first times she had been outside in months. Elaine appeared pale and frail and said she had lost about 10 pounds in recent months. I sent her to a psychiatrist to be assessed for clinical depression, and he referred her to a support group for COPD/emphysema sufferers. Through that program, Elaine increased her level of activity with scheduled daily walks in the park, tai chi classes, and emphysema-specific breathing exercises, which didn't trigger coughing attacks as she had feared. She later told me that many members of the group struggled with similar fatigue, and she found a great sense of comfort and camaraderie among them. After 6 months, she had gained 5 pounds of muscle mass and reported a 50 percent increase in her energy levels.

LIVER DISEASES

A healthy liver is essential for bodily functions many of us are unaware of. Besides metabolizing (breaking down) alcohol and many drugs, the liver regulates the composition of the blood, including how much sugar, protein, and fat enter the bloodstream. It removes bilirubin, a yellowish waste product that comes from the breakdown of red blood cells, and other toxins from the blood. It processes many of the nutrients that are absorbed by the intestines during the digestive process and converts those nutrients into usable forms for the body. It also produces cholesterol, important proteins (such as albumin), and clotting factors. Various diseases and disorders impair the liver's ability to perform these functions—and lead to substantial fatigue as a result. These include alcohol abuse, infections (such as hepatitis), liver cancer, primary sclerosing cholangitis (which is more common in men), and many others.

One of the most common liver diseases I see among women is nonalcoholic fatty liver disease, which can result in two different disease processes: a simple accumulation of fat in the liver or nonalcoholic steatohepatitis (NASH), in which there is fat accumulation and damage to the liver cells and scarring of the liver (aka cirrhosis). With NASH, liver inflammation is caused by a buildup of fat in the liver. For some people, the condition doesn't cause symptoms, but for others, NASH turns out to be a hidden cause of fatigue (as well as weight loss, weakness, and mild pain in the upper right quadrant of the abdomen). The disease doesn't always progress in severity, but when it does, NASH is similar to the kind of liver disease that is caused by long-term, heavy drinking—and yet NASH occurs in people who don't abuse alcohol.

At this point, experts don't know why some people who have a buildup of fat in their livers get NASH and some don't. It could be that something in the environment triggers liver inflammation in some people, or it could be that genetics play a role. What is known is that certain factors put people at risk for NASH and for liver damage, including obesity, type 2 diabetes, high cholesterol and triglycerides, and metabolic syndrome. Most people who have NASH are between the ages of 40 and 50 and have one or more of these risk factors—but the disease also occurs in people who have none of these risk factors.

During a follow-up to a routine physical that included a battery of blood tests, Margaret, a 50-year-old museum executive, was found to have elevated liver enzymes. She hadn't complained of any symptoms during the exam, but after the lab results came back and I pressed her for details about how she'd been feeling, she mentioned that she always felt tired. She thought it was just a part of getting older and a result of her busy travel schedule. Her blood sugar was normal, and her total cholesterol was on the high side of normal, but her triglycerides were markedly elevated. Margaret was slightly overweight, and she said she "had never exercised in her life." She drank minimal alcohol.

It wasn't immediately clear why her liver enzymes might be elevated. I sent her for an ultrasound and a CT scan, which showed significant fat accumulation in the liver, consistent with NASH. At first, she was surprised by this diagnosis, but then she recalled how her grandmother had died of liver cirrhosis, which was always mystifying to her family because the grandmother didn't drink alcohol. After her own diagnosis, Margaret started a vegetarian diet and began exercising daily, and she lost 25 pounds. (Weight loss and exercise are the primary forms of treatment for NASH.) Within a year, her liver enzymes returned to the high end of the normal range, and her energy level increased dramatically.

Fatigue is also considered the worst symptom for 50 percent of people who have primary biliary cirrhosis (PBC), a progressive disease that's caused by a buildup of bile, a fluid that helps with digestion, within the liver. This results in damage to the small bile ducts that normally drain bile from the liver. Over time, this buildup of pressure destroys the bile ducts, which leads to liver cell damage. As PBC progresses and more liver cells die off, it can lead to cirrhosis and liver failure. While the exact cause of PBC is unknown, it is likely an autoimmune disease, whereby the body's immune system attacks its own cells—in this case, the bile ducts are attacked and destroyed. Women are nine times more likely than men to develop PBC, and it most often develops between the ages of 40 and 60. Genetics may play a role, since many people with PBC have a family member who also had it.

Though she was not my patient, a 54-year-old grocery store clerk named Kathleen, whom I knew from my shopping expeditions, stopped me one day to tell me about the itching she was experiencing, especially at night. She knew I was a doctor and asked if I could recommend a good cream for dry skin. As we talked, she also described severe fatigue and said she lived on Red Bull drinks for energy. Kathleen was overweight and sedentary. I suggested she try Eucerin lotion for the itching but urged her to see her doctor right away for blood tests to make sure nothing else was being missed.

About 4 months later, I asked Kathleen how she was feeling. She revealed that she had the same symptoms, plus nausea and frequent stomach upset (diarrhea); she had not been to the doctor because her insurance had lapsed. I noticed that the whites of her eyes were slightly yellow; she agreed and said she had noticed a yellow tinge that would come and go several times for a day or two in the last month. I told her that yellowing of the eyes could be a sign of a life-threatening condition and encouraged her to go to the ER. There she was diagnosed with PBC, but thankfully her liver damage was not considered severe. She started taking a medication called ursodeoxycholic acid and was encouraged to lose weight and exercise. She's still working on the exercise part of the protocol, but her energy level and other symptoms have improved in the meantime.

There is also a genetic disorder called iron overload or hemochromatosis, in which there is an excessive accumulation of iron in the body. Without treatment, that buildup of extra iron damages the liver, heart, pancreas, endocrine glands, and joints. It is one of the most common genetic disorders in the United States, especially among Caucasians. The disease isn't always identified promptly because early symptoms—such as fatigue and weakness—are similar to those of many other common diseases. The disease is often discovered when elevated iron blood levels are noted during routine blood testing. In men, symptoms may not appear until ages 40 to 50; since women lose iron when they bleed due to their monthly periods, some women don't develop symptoms of hemochromatosis until they reach menopause and stop menstruating. Severe signs and symptoms of iron overload include sexual dysfunction, heart failure, joint pain, cirrhosis of the liver, severe fatigue, and darkening of the skin.

A less common condition, Wilson's disease is an inherited disorder in which too much copper accumulates in the liver, brain, and other vital organs. While the accumulation of copper begins at birth, symptoms of the disorder don't appear until later in life. Signs and symptoms vary widely, depending on which organs are affected, but often include fatigue, poor appetite, jaundice, a tendency to bruise easily, fluid buildup in the legs or abdomen, muscle tremors or rigidity, difficulty with speech, and abrupt changes in personality, behavior, or the ability to function at work or school. Wilson's disease is diagnosed through blood and urine tests (to check copper levels) and an eye exam to look for a deep copper-colored ring around the edge of the cornea (what's called a Kayser-Fleischer ring, a diagnostic feature of Wilson's that's caused by copper deposits in the eye). The primary form of treatment is a drug called penicillamine, a chelating agent that causes the organs to release copper into the bloodstream so it can be excreted through urine.

Two years ago, a 20-year-old college student named Maya, who lived with her family in my building, began struggling in her classes after being a straight-A student in high school. During her first year at an Ivy League college, her grades dropped dramatically, Maya lost her ability to focus, and she started sleeping all the time. She was diagnosed with depression at her school health clinic, and she was started on an antidepressant. She may well have been depressed, but I suspected there was another underlying issue going on as well because of the dramatic change in her demeanor.

Maya took a semester off and came to see me in the office for medical clearance to return to school (I had not seen her as a patient before; her pediatrician had handled her precollege screenings). When I asked how she was feeling, Maya reported that her debilitating fatigue had not resolved, and her ability to concentrate had not improved either; also, she had recently lost 10 pounds without trying. Lab work showed slightly elevated liver enzymes, which prompted me to order more extensive blood work and refer her to a specialist, who diagnosed her with Wilson's disease. Maya was given penicillamine, and her fatigue, foggy mind, and depressive symptoms resolved completely.

Another liver disease linked with debilitating fatigue is hepatitis, which is basically inflammation of the liver. The majority of hepatitis cases are caused by viruses, including hepatitis A, which is most commonly transmitted in contaminated drinking water or food; hepatitis B, which is transmitted through sexual contact, exposure to contaminated blood, and from mother to child during pregnancy; and hepatitis C, which is spread most readily through exposure to infected blood (intravenous drugs are the most common mode of transmission).

Besides fatigue, each of these illnesses has several symptoms in common (these include fever, yellowish skin and eyes, nausea, joint pain, and sore muscles), and each carries an increased risk of developing cirrhosis and liver failure. Hepatitis B infection occurs subtly and gradually, usually over several decades; as with hepatitis C, one of the earliest signs of hepatitis B is fatigue and a general feeling of being unwell, but many people disregard these as normal signs of aging.

Blood tests can diagnose all three forms of viral hepatitis. Types B and C are typically treated with antiviral medications (such as interferon); depending on the severity or duration of the illness, liver function tests or biopsies are sometimes recommended to assess long-term damage. Fortunately, two of these can be prevented now that there are vaccines for hepatitis A and B; these days, children are vaccinated for hepatitis B on a routine basis.

CHRONIC KIDNEY DISEASE

Chronic kidney disease (aka chronic renal insufficiency) can be an insidious condition that happens over the course of 20 or even 30 years. Simply put, chronic kidney disease (CKD) causes destruction of the kidneys in a gradual, progressive, irreversible fashion. Each kidney has about a million tiny structures called nephrons that are involved in the removal of waste products and excess water from the blood. If the nephrons are damaged, they stop working. For a while, healthy nephrons pick up the slack and take on the extra work, but if the damage continues, more and more nephrons shut down. After a certain point, the nephrons that remain functional cannot filter blood well enough to maintain its homeostasis (its ability to maintain a constant internal environment).

The Centers for Disease Control and Prevention estimates that 10 percent of US adults—more than 20 million people—have CKD, and the risk increases after age 50. Although routine blood tests are able to pick up the beginning of renal injury, symptoms may be mild or "nonspecific" until kidney damage becomes severe. These include fatigue, malaise, cloudy thinking, headaches, nausea or stomach upset, and poor appetite. More than 90 percent of people with CKD report suffering from lack of energy, and many feel tired after routine exertion that accompanies activities of daily living.

Anemia, a shortage of oxygen-carrying red blood cells, is often a contributing factor to the significant fatigue that's associated with CKD. A little biological background: The kidneys secrete a hormone called erythropoietin, which stimulates the bone marrow to generate red blood cells; damaged kidneys make less erythropoietin, so the red blood cell count drops and cells throughout the body may receive insufficient oxygen, thus lowering the body's energy supply. This can also happen with iron-deficiency anemia: Our bodies need iron to make hemoglobin, and when we don't have enough iron, we don't make enough hemoglobin; as the level of hemoglobin falls, your blood's ability to deliver oxygen to the brain, heart, muscles, and other tissues drops. Whatever the underlying cause is, anemia makes you feel tired, sensitive to cold, and less able to focus, and it compromises your ability to fight off illnesses and diseases.

Another factor contributing to CKD-induced fatigue: electrolyte disturbances. The kidneys regulate the extracellular fluid (the fluid outside cells) in your body and prevent that fluid from becoming too concentrated or too dilute. Without this function, electrolyte imbalances can occur—such as high potassium, low bicarbonate, low magnesium, and increased uric acid levels in the blood—which impair the cells' oxygen-carrying capacity and cause dehydration as the body tries to restore homeostasis. Fatigue is one of the most common symptoms of dehydration.

Moreover, the kidneys are responsible for clearing waste products (such as urea, which gives urine its odor) that come from the breakdown of protein from the blood: After kidney damage occurs, by-products build up, and high levels of urea can also result in high levels of ammonia in the blood. Both substances act directly on the brain to cause fatigue and poor cognition.

Angela, a 54-year-old retired teacher, came to see me because she'd been experiencing extreme fatigue for about 4 months and required 2-hour daily naps; she was also experiencing ankle swelling after being on her feet for more than 20 minutes at a time. Angela was moderately overweight, and while she didn't do formal exercise, she is an active gardener. She had been diagnosed with high blood pressure in her twenties but had never taken medications to control it, despite pleas from all of her doctors. Her reasoning: The meds cause side effects, particularly weight gain, whereas she experienced no side effects from the high blood pressure. During her office visits, her blood pressure typically ran about 150/95, which is high but definitely not a hypertensive emergency.

Because of her complaints of extreme fatigue, I ordered a battery of blood and urine tests, which showed stage 3 chronic kidney disease with mild protein loss in the urine (a sign of chronic kidney disease). Angela was given an ACE inhibitor to reduce her blood pressure, and she began following a kidney-specific form of the DASH diet, which helped her lose 20 pounds. (Dietary Approaches to Stop Hypertension, or DASH, relies on reducing sodium and eating plenty of whole grains, vegetables, fruits, and low-fat dairy products that are rich in nutrients like potassium, calcium, and magnesium that help lower blood pressure.) Thanks to these interventions, the protein in Angela's urine disappeared, and her symptoms of fatigue lessened.

The most common causes of CKD are high blood pressure and diabetes, both of which damage the nephrons, the kidneys' functional units. High blood pressure can also damage the blood vessels of the kidneys, heart, and brain. Other causes of CKD include glomerulonephritis (inflammation of the glomeruli—the kidneys' filtering units—caused by lupus or a strep infection); interstitial nephritis (inflammation of the kidneys' tubules and surrounding structures, caused most often by lupus, sarcoidosis, and abuse of nonsteroidal anti-inflammatory drugs, or NSAIDs, like celecoxib and ibuprofen); polycystic kidney disease (an inherited disorder in which clusters of noncancerous, fluid-filled cysts develop primarily within the kidneys and cause high blood pressure and kidney disease); prolonged obstruction of the urinary tract (from kidney stones and some cancers); vesicoureteral reflux (a condition that causes urine to back up into the kidneys); and recurrent kidney infections.

CKD is diagnosed with a blood test to measure the glomerular filtration rate and determine the stage of the disease (there are five). In addition, your doctor may recommend having an ultrasound, a CT scan, or an MRI of your kidneys to assess their structure and size; a biopsy of tissue from the kidney also may be warranted to help determine what's causing the disease. Treatment generally focuses on managing the underlying cause of the disease (such as high blood pressure or type 2 diabetes) and complications of CKD such as fluid retention, anemia, brittle bones, and electrolyte imbalances.

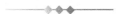

As you can see, there are many different mechanisms through which organ dysfunction leads to fatigue. Your heart, lungs, kidneys, and liver are considered vital organs for a good reason: They are essential to life, health, energy, and overall well-being. When your heart pumps efficiently and promotes steady bloodflow throughout your body, when your lungs bring in plenty of oxygen and eliminate carbon dioxide, when your kidneys and liver remove waste products and toxins from your blood and maintain the proper fluid balance in your body, you are able to maintain homeostasis, the optimal state of equilibrium for your body. When one of these organ systems goes out of whack, functional imbalances occur that drain your energy. If, based on your symptoms (you'll find a comprehensive checklist in Chapter 14), you suspect one of your organs isn't operating the way it should, see your doctor. Getting the right diagnosis and treatment can improve your fatigue and other symptoms, reduce the risk of complications from the disease—and quite possibly save your life.

CHAPTER TEN

It's a Gut Feeling: Gastrointestinal Disorders

All disease begins in the gut.
–Hippocrates, the father of medicine

IF YOU'VE EVER HAD a nasty stomach bug or a bad bout of food poisoning, you are all too familiar with how utterly depleted a gastrointestinal problem can make you feel. So imagine if that kind of digestive distress were chronic or recurring: You'd probably feel weak and wiped out, like a mere shadow of yourself, on a regular basis. Yet you might take steps to hide it since it can be hard to discuss digestive difficulties in polite company. But there's really no need to suffer in silence, because many disorders such as Crohn's disease, celiac disease, inflammatory bowel disease, and irritable bowel syndrome, as well as peptic ulcers and gastroesophageal reflux, are highly treatable.

All of the major gastrointestinal disorders, and even minor digestive imbalances, count fatigue as one of their primary presenting symptoms. The fatigue in this context has many different causes—bacterial balances in the gut, nutrient absorption issues, inflammation, sleep disturbances, and medications that are used to treat these disorders, among other factors. To understand how profoundly gastrointestinal disorders can affect your energy and vitality, it helps to have a little biological background: Our intestine (or gut, if you prefer) is often appropriately referred to as our second brain. Those 30 feet of intestinal loops contain an intricate network of 100 million neurons embedded in their lining, nearly as many as the brain, and they function independently.

In fact, the nervous system in your belly does a lot more than just break down and absorb the food you eat. It has nerve fibers that carry messages from your gastrointestinal (GI) tract to your brain, and it churns out neurotransmitters—such as dopamine and serotonin—that are normally associated with the brain in your head. It may shock you to learn that 95 percent of the feel-good neurotransmitter serotonin that's produced in your body comes from your gut, not your brain. This means that when your gastrointestinal tract isn't functioning properly, your mood often takes a hit along with your energy. Not surprisingly, in a study involving 399 patients at an outpatient GI clinic in Göteborg, Sweden, and 399 age- and gender-matched controls, researchers found that people with chronic GI diseases had more severe fatigue, poorer overall psychological well-being, and more sleep disturbances than their peers who were free of GI problems.

We've long known that the gut and brain communicate: When you feel anxious or upset, for example, you may feel it in your gut as butterflies in your stomach, nausea, or diarrhea. But now we understand that if your gut is upset—if your digestive system isn't functioning optimally, in other words—you may feel it in your brain as fatigue, anxiety, depression, or other mood disturbances.

Just as bacteria in the gut can influence your brain and behavior, your brain can have powerful effects on the bacteria that are teeming in your gut. It's a busy two-way street indeed. Research has found that psychological stress suppresses beneficial bacteria in the gut, which makes you more vulnerable to infectious diseases; these changes to the gut bacteria in turn affect brain function (including learning and memory), mood, and behavior.

The proper functioning of the GI tract depends, in part, on having the optimal balance of good and bad bacteria. Believe it or not, your gut is home to a community of hundreds of trillions of bacteria from more than 400 species—this is collectively known as the microbiome. And that's a good thing, because good bacteria aid our digestion, gut motility, and nutrient absorption; they also play a role in the removal of toxins and are thought to communicate directly with neurons in the gut that ultimately affect our mood and energy levels. Beneficial bacteria boost our immune function, promote good health and vitality, and produce neurochemicals the brain uses to regulate physiological processes (such as sleep, appetite, and sexuality) and mental processes (like learning, memory, and mood).

Beneficial bacteria can also prevent the (over)growth of harmful bacteria that make us sick and tired. Studies in animals have even found that tinkering with the proportion of good to bad bacteria in the gut alters brain chemistry in ways that affect mood and behavior. But these good bacteria are arguably under attack in our modern-day environment. Antibiotics wreak havoc on the gut because they kill both good and bad bacteria. Even if you haven't taken antibiotics in ages, you're likely still exposed because the meat and animal products we consume have been exposed to antibiotics, and our soaps, cleaning supplies, hand sanitizers, and even some tissues are laced with "antibacterial" chemicals. Other "good bacteria" killers are medicines like antacids and anti-inflammatory medicines. So the foods you eat and the medications you take, along with other aspects of your lifestyle, influence the types of bacteria that take up residence in your gut.

It's not just the state of your microbiome that influences how your GI tract affects you in the energy-versus-exhaustion equation. Various GI disorders trigger significant fatigue in a number of ways, yet almost all of them affect our ability to maximize the nutritional impact of our diet. During my first year of medical school, one of my professors memorably opened a lecture by saying, "It's possible for your mouth to follow the perfect diet, and for your cells to be starving." And it's true! What you eat is vital to good health, but how it's digested, absorbed, and eliminated is even more important.

Getting nutrients where they need to go in your body requires a perfect synchrony of steps by multiple organs; gastrointestinal disorders like Crohn's disease and other inflammatory bowel diseases (IBDs) compromise the intestine's ability to fully digest nutrients by affecting enzymes that are necessary

The Power of Probiotics

Since the beneficial bacteria in your gut have such a positive effect on your digestive health and overall sense of well-being, it stands to reason that it would be wise to add more good bacteria to your life. Research studies suggest that probiotic supplements—such as those containing beneficial bacteria strains such as *Lactobacillus acidophilus, L. casei, L. reuteri, L. rhamnosus,* and *Bifidobacterium*—improve mood and lower stress hormone levels and may help serious mental-health conditions like obsessive-compulsive disorder and schizoaffective disorder. And a large pilot study found that probiotic supplements eased anxiety and depression in patients with chronic fatigue syndrome. I'm not quite ready to recommend that everyone start taking probiotic supplements, but I may be someday.

In the meantime, if you have a particular health condition like irritable bowel syndrome or constipation, ask your doctor whether you might benefit from consuming particular probiotic strains. If you want to bolster your health and energy in general, it can't hurt and it just might help to consume probiotics from foods such as yogurt, kefir, acidophilus milk, tempeh, aged cheeses, and fortified juices and soy beverages. After all, research suggests that probiotics ward off intestinal infections (such as traveler's diarrhea and foodborne illnesses), alleviate diarrhea that stems from antibiotics, prevent stomach ulcers, and improve irritable bowel syndrome. Consuming a probiotic food per day might help keep digestive distress at bay.

for absorption (such as intrinsic factor and vitamin B_{12}, for example) or by eliminating foods before digestion has had the chance to be completed (because of frequent diarrhea, for instance). As a result, the cells in your body become undernourished, and they are unable to produce energy, which leaves you feeling tired.

The inflammation that's associated with many of these conditions is believed to cause fatigue on a chemical level. With irritable bowel syndrome (IBS), for example, scientists theorize that an immune response in the gut triggers changes in the secretion of digestive enzymes or the way the bowel moves or senses pain. This immune response could then stimulate the production of inflammatory substances that cause fatigue. Other GI disorders, including IBD (ulcerative colitis, in particular), are characterized by inflammation in a particular part of the intestines, which could partly explain the fatigue associated with these conditions. The inflammation may lead to overstimulation of the immune system; damage to mitochondria (the batteries within our cells); and the promotion of oxidative stress, including the formation of cell-damaging free radicals (which interfere with the delivery of oxygen and nutrients to the cells). Inflammation also triggers the stress response system in the brain, and as we've already seen in Chapter 4, the chronic effects of stress hormones like cortisol can deplete a person's energy over time.

In addition, medications that are used to treat certain chronic GI disorders can sap your energy. Histamine (H2) blockers and proton pump inhibitors (PPIs), which are both used to treat gastroesophageal reflux disease, directly cause fatigue. Moreover, PPIs may reduce stomach acid production so dramatically that your intestine can't absorb iron and vitamin B_{12} from food, which leads to anemia and hence fatigue. By itself, gastroesophageal reflux disease can also cause sleep disruptions—thanks to the discomfort or coughing that stems from having the contents of your stomach flow into your esophagus while you're lying down—which leave you feeling wrecked in the morning. Moreover, anxiety, depression, and sleep difficulties often accompany Crohn's disease, ulcerative colitis, and IBS, which result in a constant state of depletion.

The bottom line: If you're tired, it's worth taking a long, hard look at your gut health. It may hold the key to a remedy for your exhaustion. What follows is a guide to the signs and symptoms of some of the most common chronic digestive disorders that can cause fatigue.

CELIAC DISEASE

When people with celiac disease (aka celiac sprue) consume gluten (a protein that's found in wheat, rye, and barley), their bodies trigger an immune reaction that attacks the small intestine and leads to damage on the villi (tiny, fingerlike projections on the lining of the intestinal wall). When the villi are damaged, nutrients from food can't be absorbed properly. Besides being a disease of malabsorption, celiac disease involves an abnormal immune response to gluten. Symptoms vary considerably but often include abdominal bloating and pain, chronic diarrhea, vomiting, gas and flatulence, pale stools, and fatigue. Celiac disease can lead to iron-deficiency anemia, which worsens fatigue, as well as depression or anxiety, bone or joint pain, or an itchy skin rash called dermatitis herpetiformis.

Celiac disease affects at least three million people in the United States, and many other cases are undiagnosed. The average time from the onset of symptoms to diagnosis is 4 years. While the exact cause is unknown, the disease tends to cluster in families: People who have a first-degree relative with celiac disease (a parent, child, or sibling) have a 1 in 10 risk of developing celiac disease themselves. Women are affected more often than men are, and the disorder is most common in Caucasians and people of European ancestry.

Celiac disease can develop at any age after people start eating foods or medicines that contain gluten. Research suggests that the later the age of diagnosis, the greater the person's chances are of developing another autoimmune disorder such as Addison's disease, Crohn's disease, multiple sclerosis, or Sjögren's syndrome. Left untreated, celiac disease causes additional serious health problems, such as osteoporosis, infertility and miscarriage, neurological conditions like epilepsy and migraines, and intestinal cancers and lymphoma.

To diagnose the condition, doctors will order initial blood tests to check for high levels of anti-tissue transglutaminase antibodies and anti-immunoglobulin A antibodies. If blood test results and your symptoms suggest celiac disease, a biopsy of the small intestine is performed: A tiny piece of tissue is removed to check for damage to the villi, to confirm the diagnosis. Treatment is simple: strict gluten avoidance (aka a gluten-free diet) for life. This resolves symptoms in nearly all sufferers.

When Amy, a 28-year-old graphic designer, came in for a routine physical a few years ago, she asked for a referral to a dermatologist because she had an annoying rash on the backs of her elbows. The rash had come and gone since her teen years, but it had recently worsened and would occasionally bleed and get crusty. When I asked her about other symptoms and her lifestyle habits, she told me she was drinking six to eight cups of coffee during the day to stay energized, and she would sleep for most of the weekend. She also mentioned that when she went out on dates, she would avoid eating because her stomach would visibly expand and look downright large, which embarrassed her. Once I heard these details, I ordered blood tests for celiac autoantibodies, which came back positive. Amy didn't want to have a biopsy to confirm the diagnosis; instead, she began adhering to a strict gluten-free diet, which resolved all her symptoms.

IRRITABLE BOWEL SYNDROME

If the name makes you think of cranky intestines, you're on the right track. Irritable bowel syndrome (IBS) is a common disorder (not a disease) of the intestines that leads to abdominal cramping and pain, gas, bloating, alternating bouts of diarrhea and constipation, and mucus in the stool. An estimated 10 to 20 percent of adults in the United States suffer from IBS, and it's twice as prevalent among women. It's also present in about 80 percent of people with chronic fatigue syndrome and unexpectedly high among people with anxiety disorders.

While the cause isn't known, IBS is considered a functional disorder because the symptoms stem from an oversensitivity of the muscles, nerves, and intestine, which affects the way they function. There are no structural abnormalities, and IBS doesn't cause permanent harm to the intestine. But people with IBS can experience a great deal of discomfort, which is almost always exhausting. Since there isn't a test for IBS, the diagnosis is made largely on the basis of a person's symptoms but may include an abdominal x-ray, stool cultures, and/or colonoscopy or sigmoidoscopy to rule out other GI disorders.

When I first saw Isabella, a 19-year-old college student who gets straight A's, she told me she'd always had a "sensitive stomach," with bouts of gas and bloating after large meals. She had recently begun experiencing explosive diarrhea, occasionally with episodes of incontinence in public. After having diarrhea, she would be constipated for several days. She felt exhausted but too anxious to sleep well. Once we ruled out other disorders, I diagnosed her with IBS and she began taking a tricyclic antidepressant, which resolved her diarrhea but didn't completely eliminate her persistent fatigue. She's now trying other approaches—including dietary modifications and meditation—to boost her energy.

If specific dietary triggers can be identified (common ones include gluten, lactose, and gas-producing vegetables like Brussels sprouts and beans), patients are usually advised to avoid them. For many people, sticking with a healthy diet—including consuming plenty of fiber to bulk up stools and keep things moving smoothly through the GI tract and probiotics (see "The Power of Probiotics" on page 140)—and avoiding large quantities of food at any given time reduce symptoms. A variety of medications, including antidepressants, antispasmodics, antidiarrheals, laxatives, and others, are also available. IBS often flares up when people are under stress, and natural interventions like cognitive behavioral therapy and meditation have been shown to reduce the symptoms of IBS as well as the anxiety that's often associated with the condition. Ultimately, treatment is highly individualized.

GASTROESOPHAGEAL REFLUX DISEASE

Everyone experiences heartburn now and then, but for the 15 million people in the United States who experience it on a daily basis, it's a fact of life. When heartburn becomes chronic, it's called gastroesophageal reflux disease (GERD), which occurs when the stomach contents and acid flow up into your lower esophagus. This backwash is due to a weakening or excessive relaxing of the lower esophageal sphincter, a muscle that acts as a valve between the stomach and the esophagus. GERD affects people of all ages, but the risk increases during pregnancy or if you smoke, you're obese, or you have a hiatal hernia.

Heartburn is the most common symptom; others include a dry cough, chest pain, and a recurrent sore throat. Constant fatigue develops for several reasons: GERD can disturb sleep; severe GERD causes bleeding in the lower esophagus, which can lead to anemia and fatigue; and some of the medications that are used to treat GERD, such as H2 blockers and proton pump inhibitors, cause tiredness in some people (they also interfere with the absorption of vitamin B$_{12}$, which can lead to fatigue).

A few years ago, my friend Victoria, then 30, was complaining of bronchitis that she just couldn't kick. She mentioned constantly clearing her throat (most dramatically in the morning) and that she had a dry cough all day. She was a heavy smoker (two packs a day), and she took nonsteroidal anti-inflammatory drugs for headaches daily. When I asked, she said she didn't have chest pain or heartburn symptoms, but she said she was more tired than she'd ever been, even though she was sleeping her usual amount.

I sent her for an endoscopy, a test that involves passing a small, lighted, flexible tube through the mouth and into the esophagus and stomach to look for abnormalities. (Sometimes blood tests and breath tests for specific bacteria or a pH probe to test for the presence of acid in the upper GI tract are used to diagnose GERD, but these weren't necessary in Victoria's case.) Sure enough, she had severe gastritis (inflammation of the stomach lining) and erosive esophagitis (inflammation in the esophagus), both complications of GERD. I treated her with H2 blockers and encouraged her to stop smoking and stop taking NSAIDs so frequently. Unfortunately, she hasn't been able to ditch the smoking habit, but she did quit NSAIDs and feels much less tired these days. The dry cough and throat clearing were resolved, too.

Treatment of GERD often involves other medications (such as PPIs) and lifestyle changes (such as avoiding alcohol, fatty foods, and other triggers like citrus juice, tomato juice, spicy foods, and chocolate) that may irritate an already irritated esophagus. GERD sufferers should avoid eating for 2 hours before bedtime and raise the head of their beds with a foam wedge to elevate the head and prevent reflux symptoms during sleep. If obesity is contributing to the problem, weight loss helps. In extreme cases, surgery to strengthen the lower esophageal sphincter may be an option. One way or another, it's important to get GERD symptoms under good control—for the sake of your current and future well-being. Left untreated, GERD may lead to complications such as Barrett's esophagus (a precancerous condition) and esophageal cancer.

INFLAMMATORY BOWEL DISEASE

This is an umbrella term for two different diseases: ulcerative colitis and Crohn's disease, which have overlapping symptoms, including fatigue. In a 2014 study, researchers from Italy found that patients with IBD who had moderate to severe disease activity had worse fatigue compared to their healthy peers at every age; even those whose disease was in remission had severe fatigue. The causes of IBD aren't known, but it does tend to run in families. Up to 30 percent of people with IBD have a relative with the condition. Despite having the familial and fatigue factors in common, Crohn's disease and ulcerative colitis are distinct entities. Here's how they compare.

Crohn's Disease

A chronic disease that has periods of remission, Crohn's causes inflammation and ulceration deep in the intestinal wall and sometimes in other parts of the GI tract. The age of onset is usually between 15 and 40, and it occurs slightly more often in women. Common symptoms include abdominal pain and cramping, diarrhea, blood in the stool, weight loss, fever, mouth sores, and fatigue.

Since there isn't a single test for Crohn's disease, your doctor may use a combination of blood tests, endoscopy, and radiologic testing (such as colonoscopy, CT scans, or MRI scans) to make the diagnosis. Treatment involves medications to reduce inflammation (corticosteroids, immunosuppressants, and others) and prevent long-term complications; sometimes surgery is performed to remove damaged parts of the digestive tract.

Ulcerative Colitis

In some ways, this type of IBD is similar to Crohn's—similar age of onset, similar family history, similar diagnostic methods—but ulcerative colitis usually affects only the innermost lining of the large intestine (the colon) and the rectum. Symptoms—such as diarrhea (often with blood or pus), abdominal pain and cramping, rectal pain and bleeding, weight loss, fatigue, and fever—usually develop over time, not suddenly. Besides being debilitating, ulcerative colitis can lead to serious complications such as anemia, osteoporosis, a perforated colon, an increased risk of blood clots, and an increased risk of colon cancer.

There isn't a cure, but treatment significantly reduces symptoms of the disease. Commonly used medications include anti-inflammatory drugs, corticosteroids, and immunosuppressants. In some cases, surgery is an option: It can ultimately cure the disease, but it usually means removing the entire colon and rectum, which is major surgery.

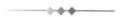

It's a mistake to ignore digestive woes, for the sake of your overall health and well-being as well as your energy and vitality. If you have symptoms that suggest you have a chronic gastrointestinal disorder, trust your gut instincts: Take an inventory of your symptoms (using the checklist in Chapter 14) and schedule a visit with your physician to go over them. To prepare for the appointment, it helps to keep a diary (see Appendix A for a template) in which you keep track of everything you put in your mouth (and the time), as well as your sleep schedule, and how your symptoms vary throughout the day and night. In the meantime, sticking with a nutrient-rich diet (including plenty of fluids and plant-based foods that are high in fiber), regular physical activity, sufficient sleep, and good stress-management practices—all part of your personalized energy-boosting plan—can help you start to feel better. These healthy lifestyle factors may even ease your digestive troubles and get your GI system running more smoothly, which will start you on the road to recovery.

CHAPTER ELEVEN

Hostile Takeovers: Infections

WHEN YOU'RE SICK WITH a fever, body aches, chills, and other dramatic symptoms, you probably expect to feel weak, tired, and lethargic because you're undeniably ill. But often the signs of an infection are subtle, in which case it's not as easy to connect the dots between your fatigue or lackluster energy and the possibility that your body is fighting an infection. Since the dawn of time, infectious agents have been ubiquitous in this world, and countless people contract infections ranging from garden-variety sinus or urinary tract infections to more serious illnesses such as mononucleosis, influenza (the flu), or HIV (the human immunodeficiency virus, which causes AIDS). To varying degrees, infections tax the immune system and trigger inflammation, which can leave you feeling mildly worn out or utterly spent. Indeed, numerous studies have found that chronically fatigued people have higher blood markers of inflammation such as C-reactive protein and proinflammatory compounds called cytokines.

It has long been believed that the fatigue and malaise we experience when we're fighting an infection is an evolutionary survival mechanism—one that's designed to make us slow down and rest so that our bodies can focus their energy on winning the battle against the bacteria, virus, or other agent that's making us sick or threatening our health. And this may be as good an explanation as any. After all, when your immune system is busy mounting a full-throttle attack on the germs that are making you ill, energy and resources are diverted away from giving you the get-up-and-go to perform daily activities at an optimal level. (That's why it's important to heed your body's fatigue signals when you're sick and to rest rather than push yourself to power through your usual responsibilities.)

On a physiological level, there may be more specific ways infections cause fatigue. One of the most significant involves the inflammatory response: During the earliest stages of an infection, when immune defenses are activated, cytokines (proteins that act as messengers between cells) are produced in abundance. More than 80 known cytokines—including various interferons, TNF (tumor necrosis factor), and numerous interleukins—are secreted by infected cells. The rapid release of these cytokines at the site of infection initiates the release of other immune cells that have far-reaching consequences—including inflammation, which is associated with fatigue. Moreover, when cytokines enter the bloodstream, they can cause fever, sleepiness, lethargy, muscle pain, loss of appetite, and nausea. A vicious cycle may begin when the infection-induced fatigue persists, which further weakens your defenses and leaves you more vulnerable to new infections.

You don't, however, have to be super-sick or in the later stages of an infectious disease to feel wiped out; even low-grade infections can sap your energy and leave you exhausted. If you've ever had a urinary tract infection (UTI), you're probably familiar with the burning pain and sense of urgency that accompanies your trips to the bathroom. But the infection does not always announce itself with such obvious symptoms. In some cases, fatigue may be the primary sign.

Not long ago, Tanya, a 37-year-old mother at my daughter's nursery school, asked me for a referral to a specialist in autoimmune disorders because she had been experiencing severe fatigue and lethargy for about 6 months. Tanya had recently had another baby, and her primary-care physician suggested she might be suffering from postpartum depression and referred her to a psychiatrist. The psychiatrist determined that Tanya was not depressed, but her fatigue didn't budge. After extensive Google searches, she became convinced she had some sort of autoimmune disorder or chronic fatigue syndrome. She knew that these disorders tend to cluster in families, and her younger sister had recently been diagnosed with lupus.

I gave Tanya the name of a rheumatologist to whom I frequently refer patients. A few weeks later, she told me the doctor had done urine testing during her battery of tests that showed an active and severe urinary tract infection; a follow-up ultrasound discovered scarring of one of her kidneys, scarring that's consistent with chronic or recurrent kidney infections (pyelo-nephritis). After a 10-day course of antibiotics, Tanya's fatigue disappeared and she regained her former energy. Her experience is noteworthy because she hadn't experienced burning or frequency of urination or back pain—the classic symptoms of an entrenched UTI or kidney infection.

The take-home message: It's a mistake to overlook the possibility of infection if you have long-standing fatigue even in the absence of obvious symptoms. What follows is a look at some of the sneakier infections that can drain your energy and leave you exhausted.

CHRONIC FATIGUE SYNDROME

Chronic fatigue syndrome is a perplexing phenomenon—and one with which I'm personally familiar. I was diagnosed with overlapping chronic fatigue syndrome and fibromyalgia during medical school, and in my case, the symptoms waxed and waned: I'd have a couple of truly exhausted months and then a few months when I'd feel better. During the worst periods, I'd get up in the morning, usually 2 hours later than I'd planned to, feeling unre-freshed after a full night's sleep. I'd have 2 to 3 good, productive hours, and then I'd be dragging for the rest of the day. It wasn't the kind of fatigue that a person would normally feel at the end of the day; it was an overwhelming exhaustion and sleepiness that felt almost like being drugged.

The condition's name may not sound like it's related to an infection, so you might wonder why I'm addressing it in this chapter. While the underlying cause of chronic fatigue syndrome (CFS) isn't well understood, it may have multiple triggers, including viruses or other infections, genetic factors, brain abnormalities, an overreactive immune system, psychological or emotional conditions, and stress-related hormonal abnormalities. While CFS occurs in both sexes, at all ages, and in all racial and ethnic groups, women are more likely to be diagnosed with it than men. The Centers for Disease Control and Prevention estimates that more than 1 million people in the United States have CFS, and millions more have similar symptoms but do not meet the full criteria for a CFS diagnosis.

Chronic fatigue syndrome is not a new disorder, but it is an increasingly recognized one. In the 19th century, the term *neurasthenia,* or nervous exhaustion, was applied to symptoms resembling those in CFS. But our view of the syndrome has evolved, and it is now recognized as a significantly debilitating medical condition. It is marked by unexplained, continuing, or returning fatigue that is either new or that started at a definite point in time, along with other specific symptoms that last for a minimum of 6 months in adults. The fatigue is not due to exertion, is not significantly relieved by rest, and is not caused by other medical conditions. But it can significantly compromise the quality of your work or school performance and your social life.

To be diagnosed with CFS, the person also must have four or more of the following symptoms on a continuous or recurring basis for 6 or more consecutive months (and the symptoms must not predate the fatigue): significant impairment in short-term memory or concentration; sore throat; tender lymph nodes; muscle pain; joint pain without swelling or redness; headaches that are new, more severe, or that occur in a different pattern than previously; unrefreshing sleep; or general discomfort or malaise that lasts for more than 24 hours after exertion. Beyond the scope of these criteria, people with CFS often have cognitive difficulties (such as challenges with finding the right words, planning ahead, and getting organized), dizziness or nausea, general malaise or flulike symptoms (that aren't caused by an infection), rapid heart-beat (palpitations) without underlying heart problems, and a worsening of symptoms with physical exertion.

Most patients with CFS report having a moderate to serious physical illness (such as a long-term viral infection) or an emotional event (like an episode of depression) before they developed CFS. Some experts believe that these factors, alone or in combination, may interact with abnormalities in the nervous system or gene abnormalities to trigger CFS. On the infection front, various types have been studied to determine if they might cause or trigger CFS. These include the Epstein-Barr virus, herpes virus 6 (which is more common among those with impaired immune systems or who take immunosuppressant drugs), entero-virus (a frequent cause of the common cold that enters through the gastroin-testinal tract), rubella (aka the German measles), and *Candida albicans* (a fungus that causes yeast infections), among others. One hypothesis is that a viral infection or stress may lead to the chronic production of cytokines and then to CFS.

The central nervous system plays an important role in CFS. Physical or emotional stress, which occurs before the onset of CFS in many people, alters the activity of the hypothalamic–pituitary–adrenal axis, leading to changes in the release of corticotropin-releasing hormone, cortisol, and other hormones. All of these hormones influence the immune system as well as many other body systems. Hormonal abnormalities also may come into play. Some CFS patients produce lower levels of cortisol than healthy people. This is significant, because cortisol suppresses inflammation and cellular immune activation, so reduced levels of cortisol might lead to excess inflam-mation and potentially a flare-up of CFS symptoms.

Allergic diseases—such as food allergies, seasonal allergies, and eczema—as well as secondary illnesses such as sinusitis also seem to predispose some people to CFS. But not all CFS sufferers have allergies or sinus problems. Many CFS patients do, however, report intolerances for certain substances such as preservatives and other additives found in foods or over-the-counter medications (such as alcohol or dyes).

Meanwhile, there is some evidence that stress triggers CFS in people who are at risk for the condition due to genetic factors. For example, people who experienced trauma during childhood, including sexual and emotional abuse, are significantly more likely to develop CFS than those who didn't experience such trauma. Researchers speculate that the stress of abuse may have effects on the central nervous system, the immune system, and the neuroendocrine system (which involves both nerves and hormones) that trigger the condition.

Another factor thought to contribute to the onset of CFS: abnormally low blood pressure. Some people with CFS have disturbances in the autonomic regulation of their blood pressure and pulse, a problem that can be diagnosed by using tilt table testing. This involves having you lie on a table that moves from a horizontal position to a vertical position (straps hold your body in place) while your blood pressure and heart rate are monitored. Under these conditions, people with neurally mediated hypotension—which involves miscommunication between the heart and the brain (instead of telling the heart to beat faster to prevent fainting, the brain erroneously tells the heart to slow down)—or orthostatic hypotension (aka postural hypotension)—a condition in which moving from lying on your back to being in an upright position causes an abnormally large increase in heart rate—will develop lower blood pressure, as well as other characteristic symptoms such as light-headedness, visual dimming, or a slow response to verbal stimuli. Many people with CFS experience light-headedness or worsened fatigue when they stand for prolonged periods of time or when they're in warm places such as a hot shower—these are symptoms of orthostatic hypotension.

Meanwhile, many CFS sufferers also have fibromyalgia, "multiple chemical sensitivity," or both. It isn't clear whether these are risk factors or direct causes, or whether they have common triggers or simply coexist by coincidence. But there are some interesting factors that overlap. For example, because fibromyalgia causes prolonged fatigue and widespread muscle aches, it is the disease that's most often confused with CFS. In fact, many experts believe fibromyalgia and CFS are different forms of the same condition. But while CFS patients experience severe fatigue, fibromyalgia patients experience more pain. People with fibromyalgia (which you'll read more about in Chapter 12) have at least 11 tender points, sites that are very sensitive and painful when touched firmly; these are often on the side of the neck, the top of the shoulder blades, outside the upper buttock and hip joint, and on the inside of the knee. Some people with CFS have similar tender pressure points. The connection between the two conditions may have to do with an increased response to stimulation (called central sensitization), which is thought to cause fibromyalgia and may also contribute to CFS.

Unfortunately, there is no proven cure for CFS, and no drug has been developed specifically for this disorder. Because CFS remains poorly understood, many patients have problems finding good care. Overall, the recommended strategy for treatment includes a combination of the following: a healthy diet, antidepressant drugs (usually low-dose tricyclic antidepressants), cognitive behavioral therapy, graded exercise therapy (a CFS-specific physical activity plan that starts very slowly and gradually increases over time) followed by a gradual return to moderate-intensity exercise, sleep management techniques, and other medications (such as nonsteroidal anti-inflammatory drugs or stimulants).

The severity of chronic fatigue syndrome varies considerably. Some people have mild cases. Others have trouble fulfilling home and work responsibilities: They cannot work more than part-time, and they have difficulty doing even simple tasks such as light housework. That's what happened to Jeannie, a 40-year-old computer programmer, who was referred to me a few years ago by her psychiatrist. For 4 years, she had been suffering from such extreme fatigue that she struggled to get out of bed and ended up losing her job. Despite her debilitating fatigue, she had trouble sleeping and would frequently awaken during the night.

Not surprisingly, Jeannie had mental fogginess and major depression during her daytime hours; she was being treated with antidepressants and therapy and reported a minimal improvement from the meds. But if she pushed herself to get through a full workday, she would develop headaches and feel even more tired for several days afterward. Exercise made her feel better for a few hours, but then she'd feel more wiped out than before. When I asked about other symptoms, she described some muscle pain in her shoulders and neck, but she didn't have pain anywhere else. Her psychiatrist wanted me to check for underlying illnesses like anemia and thyroid disorder, so I did, and all tests yielded negative results.

I suspected Jeannie had CFS and referred her to a group of neurologists who specialize in the condition, and they confirmed my suspicions. At their recommendation, Jeannie began doing cognitive behavioral therapy, performing graded exercise therapy, and taking some dietary supplements including vitamin B_{12}, magnesium, acetyl-L-carnitine (an amino acid), and DHA/EPA (omega-3 fatty acids). When I last saw her about a year ago, she expressed appreciation for the diagnosis and referral and said that it made her feel better emotionally to know that she had an identifiable condition. She said her symptoms of fatigue were slightly better overall, but they varied from week to week and she still considered herself sick and extremely impaired by the condition.

As in Jeannie's case, even with treatment, many people do not fully recover from CFS—but some do. Although several studies have reported that more than half of patients who complain of chronic fatigue are still fatigued at 2 years, with long-term treatment other patients improve and even make a nearly complete recovery. People who stay as active as possible and try to have some control over their CFS have the best chances for improvement. That's what I've done—by continuing to work as a doctor and a TV medical correspondent, making a habit of power walking, and leading a full family and social life—but I've also learned how to honor my limits and take time for R & R when necessary.

It's important to choose a physician who thinks of CFS as a medical condition with psychiatric components rather than vice versa. You should also be wary of any doctor who recommends excessive and expensive treatments that

Multiple Chemical Sensitivity

It may sound like a subjective complaint, but multiple chemical sensitivity (aka "environmental illness" or "sick building syndrome") is a real phenomenon. It occurs when people experience a variety of symptoms—such as fatigue, headache, dizziness, nausea, congestion, itching, sneezing, sore throat, breathing problems, muscle pain, digestive distress, or mood or memory changes—after being exposed to chemicals or perfumes at work or home or a major event like a chemical spill. Symptoms tend to involve more than one organ system, and they generally improve when the chemical triggers are eliminated.

What's particularly baffling is that some symptoms of multiple chemical sensitivity (MCS) are similar to those of chronic fatigue syndrome (CFS); complicating matters, many people who have CFS also have MCS. Just as with CFS and fibromyalgia, there is an ongoing debate in the medical community as to whether MCS is a specific medical condition or whether it has psychological underpinnings. We may never know for sure. After all, everyone is exposed to many different chemicals on a daily basis, so it's difficult to determine whether certain chemicals are responsible for specific symptoms. Indeed, there are no reliable tests to diagnose MCS.

Here's my advice: If being around certain chemicals, perfumes, incense, or irritants (common ones include bleach, fabric softeners, air fresheners, and insecticides) seems to make your symptoms worse, avoid exposure to those environmental culprits whenever possible. Also, choose fragrance-free personal care products and cleaning products and detergents, and try to keep your home and office as clean, "green," and well ventilated as possible.

may have serious side effects and no proven benefits. Those who have severe CFS that cannot be managed with lifestyle changes and medications should ask their doctors about the possibility of participating in a local clinical trial, because there are ongoing investigations into new treatments.

EPSTEIN-BARR VIRUS

The Epstein-Barr virus (EBV) causes mononucleosis, also known as mono. It belongs to the family of herpes viruses that include those that cause cold sores, genital herpes, chicken pox, and shingles. Infection with EBV is virtually inescapable: In the United States, 50 percent of all children will be infected by age 5, and 95 percent of all adults by age 40; yet many people don't realize they have the virus because their symptoms are mild and mimic the symptoms of a run-of-the-mill cold. Once you're infected with it, however, you harbor the virus for good. There is growing concern about the after-effects of EBV, because a number of chronic diseases, including chronic fatigue syndrome and some types of cancers (such as cancer of the nasopharynx, which is the cavity behind the mouth, as well as Hodgkin's disease and non-Hodgkin's lymphoma), have been linked to this infection.

When symptoms of mononucleosis (aka EBV infection) do occur, they typically include fatigue, fever, an inflamed sore throat, swollen lymph nodes in the neck, an enlarged spleen, and liver inflammation. People who do get symptoms from EBV infection—usually teenagers or adults—generally get better in 2 to 4 weeks; however, some people may feel fatigued for months. EBV spreads most commonly through bodily fluids, especially saliva. It's much more rarely passed on through blood and semen during sexual contact, blood transfusions, and organ transplants. Sharing objects such as a toothbrush or a drink or kissing an infected person spreads the virus. The first time you are infected with EBV, you may be contagious for weeks, even before you have symptoms.

If an EBV infection is suspected, it can usually be confirmed with a blood test that detects antibodies to the virus. This is also how CFS patients often discover they've been exposed to EBV, but it's important to remember that about 90 percent of adults have antibodies that show they have a current or past EBV infection, so it's difficult to make a cause-effect connection this way. Nevertheless, EBV infection is often the precipitating event that triggers someone's chronic fatigue symptoms.

At this point, there aren't any good treatments, cures, or vaccines to prevent the spectrum of illnesses that are linked to EBV (such as mononucleosis and CFS). But that may change someday, as development of an EBV vaccine is currently under way. For now, treatment is focused on relieving symptoms of EBV—getting plenty of rest to relieve fatigue, drinking adequate fluids to stay hydrated, and taking over-the-counter pain medications to reduce aches and fever.

Not long ago, Hallie, a 30-year-old graduate student in international affairs, came to see me after being diagnosed with EBV by the student health clinic. She said she had been diagnosed with EBV more than six times in her life. She wondered if she had an underlying immune system disorder that predisposed her to the illness. Although she described having suffered from persistent fatigue for the majority of the previous 10 years, she went to her student health clinic because she had a sore throat, extremely swollen tonsils and lymph nodes in her neck, fever, and even more dramatic fatigue than usual. Her fatigue had been so bad the year before that she had taken a semester off from her studies to rest, but that didn't help.

Because my examination revealed nothing extraordinary, I referred Hallie to an immunologist to screen for rare immune system deficiencies (such as immunoglobulin A deficiency or T cell dysfunction), the results of which turned out to be negative. Nonetheless, the immunologist decided to treat her with an antiviral drug called valacyclovir, which is used in the treatment of herpes viruses 1 and 2 and shingles but is not the standard of care with EBV. After 3 weeks, Hallie said she felt better than she had since childhood: She told me her energy level had improved by 90 percent, and her other

The Postviral Slump

It's not unusual for people to experience a profound sense of fatigue after being sick with a virus. Long after the initial fever, body aches, sore throat, coughing, and sneezing should have abated, virus sufferers can still feel walloped with an enduring sense of fatigue, and they can experience a prolonged recovery.

In a 2006 study, researchers from Sydney University in Australia followed patients from the time of their acute infection with the Epstein-Barr virus over the course of a year and found that 12 percent of the participants were still suffering from disabling fatigue, musculoskeletal pain, cognitive difficulties, and mood disturbances 6 months later. The vast majority of the participants with prolonged symptoms met the criteria for chronic fatigue syndrome. More recently, in a 2014 study involving 140 people who had a history of West Nile virus infection, researchers at the Baylor College of Medicine in Houston found that 31 percent of the participants experienced prolonged fatigue 6 months after their infections.

Besides the immunological mechanisms, there also may be neurobiological, psychological, and behavioral factors that set the stage for this kind of lingering fatigue. Plus, after people are sick with a virus, they may remain more sedentary after their primary symptoms have recovered, and this lingering inactivity may lead to downturns in physical fitness and exercise tolerance, which perpetuates their fatigue. It's not uncommon for people to feel depressed in the aftermath of a major viral illness, and depression may contribute to the postinfection fatigue as well.

Gradually returning to an exercise routine or normal physical activity has been shown to boost a person's mood and sense of physical well-being. It also helps to return to a consistent sleep routine and a healthy diet. Research from Scotland suggests that increasing your intake of essential fatty acids (linoleic, gamma-linolenic, eicosapentaenoic, and docosahexaenoic acids, in particular) may significantly improve symptoms of postviral fatigue. My feeling is that consuming more of these healthy fatty acids certainly can't hurt, and it just might help—so it's worth a try.

symptoms had resolved. The immunologist theorized that the antiviral medication could have improved her symptoms by treating a different but related virus that may have been causing her fatigue but wasn't diagnosed. The important thing is that this approach helped in Hallie's case, even though she may not be out of the woods for good.

The hitch with EBV is that once you have it, you never really get rid of it. Whereas bacteria can multiply comfortably on their own in the right environment, viruses need to insert themselves into a host's cells in order to survive and thrive. After a virus takes a human cell hostage, it tries to move on and spread its influence as it continues to conquer one cell after another. Fortunately, a healthy immune system usually stops most viruses before they gain a stronghold. Upon detecting a particular virus, the immune system makes a customized antibody, and natural killer cells mount a full-throttle attack against the virus. But like other herpes viruses, EBV is shrewd and crafty, and it can find ways to evade an aggressive antibody strike. Once the virus is in your body, it stays there in a latent (inactive) state for months or years. If the virus gets reactivated, you can potentially spread EBV to other people without realizing it, even if considerable time has passed since the initial infection—but you're unlikely to get sick this time around even if you did previously.

SINUS INFECTIONS

You might think you'd know unequivocally if you had a sinus infection, but sometimes the symptoms are subtle or sneaky. In fact, research from Vanderbilt University found that extreme fatigue is a more common indicator of a sinus infection than headache or sinus pain or pressure. Other symptoms include sleep disturbances, a thick discharge from the nose or down the back of the throat, nasal blockage or significant congestion, a decreased sense of smell or taste, ear pain, aching in your upper jaw and/or teeth, a cough that may worsen at night, a lingering sore throat, bad breath, and nausea (from postnasal drip).

Chronic sinusitis and acute sinusitis have similar signs and symptoms. Acute sinusitis is a temporary infection of the sinuses that usually goes along with the common cold. Symptoms of chronic sinusitis, a condition in which the cavities around the nasal passages (sinuses) become inflamed and swollen, last much longer and often cause more profound fatigue. Some conditions can raise your risk of getting chronic sinusitis, including nasal polyps (tissue growths that block the nasal passages), allergies (which can cause inflammation that blocks your sinus passages, leading to bacterial or fungal infections), a deviated septum (a crooked wall between the nostrils that may block the sinuses), facial trauma (such as a fractured or broken bone in the face, which can cause obstruction of the sinus passages), frequent respiratory tract infections (which can cause inflammation and thickening of the nasal membranes, blocking mucus drainage and creating conditions that are ripe for the growth of bacteria), and other medical conditions (such as cystic fibrosis, gastroesophageal reflux disease, and certain immune system–related diseases that result in nasal blockages).

Sinus infections are typically diagnosed through examination and sometimes blood tests (to check white blood cell count), nasal endoscopy, CT scan, or MRI. Treatment generally involves antibiotics, saline irrigation (such as the Neti pot), decongestants, nasal steroid spray, and sometimes nonsteroidal anti-inflammatory drugs (for pain) and oral corticosteroids (to reduce inflammation).

LYME DISEASE

Lyme disease is spread by ticks but is actually caused by a form of bacteria called *Borrelia burgdorferi* that is transmitted most commonly by infected deer ticks and sometimes Western black-legged ticks, too. It takes about 36 hours for an infected tick to spread Lyme disease, so if you remove the tick before that amount of time has elapsed, you're likely to dodge the disease. The classic symptom of Lyme disease is a bull's-eye rash (a round, red rash with parts that may clear as it enlarges, resulting in a bull's-eye pattern) that typically appears 3 to 30 days after the bite. But up to 30 percent of people who are infected with Lyme disease don't get the rash. Other symptoms of Lyme disease include fatigue, fever, chills, headache, sore muscles, and joint pain. Some people who get Lyme disease are symptom-free in the early stages and don't even remember getting a tick bite. The disease is diagnosed by a blood test and treated with antibiotics (such as doxycycline or amoxicillin); treatment is most effective when the disease is caught in the early stages.

If Lyme disease remains untreated, more serious symptoms can develop over time. These include joint swelling and pain; numbness and tingling in the hands, feet, and back; weakness in the facial muscles; a relentless lack of energy; and poor memory and trouble focusing your thoughts. Up to 20 percent of people with Lyme disease have symptoms—such as muscle and joint pain, cognitive deficits, sleep disturbances, and fatigue—that last months to years after they've been treated with antibiotics. While the cause of these long-lasting symptoms—referred to as post-treatment Lyme disease syndrome (PTLDS)—isn't known, there's no evidence that they're due to ongoing infection with *B. burgdorferi*. The current thinking is that PTLDS is the result of a continuous immune response, one that continues to damage the body's tissues, even after the infection has been cleared. Regardless of the underlying cause, studies have not definitively proven that continuing antibiotic therapy for many months is helpful, and some experts believe this approach could actually be harmful—by causing antibiotic-associated side effects or complications—for people with PTLDS. Nevertheless, this approach is frequently used and offers relief for some, even if it's just a temporary or partial improvement of symptoms.

Carolyn, a 40-year-old TV makeup artist, came to me complaining of having had 3 years of severe, one-sided headaches twice a week. The pain was not relieved by migraine treatment medications or preventive meds that were prescribed by several neurologists. During the same time period, she described debilitating fatigue, always feeling sleepy and yawning; in fact, she lost her job at a local news station because she was unable to work the required 8-hour days and was frequently late because she couldn't wake up promptly in the morning. Carolyn ended up supporting herself through freelance jobs with shorter hours. She also experienced mental fogginess, confusion, forgetfulness, and generalized achiness.

Although she could not recall being bitten by a tick, I ordered a blood test for Lyme disease, based on her history of fatigue and pain. It turned out that Carolyn had multiple positive markers for both acute and chronic Lyme disease. I referred her to a Lyme disease specialist, who diagnosed her with PTLDS and started her on monthly intravenous antibiotic infusions for a year. After 6 months of treatment, she said her fatigue and aches had improved by about 80 percent, but the mental fogginess remained.

Fortunately, many people with PTLDS get better with time, but it can take many months. This doesn't mean your life has to come to a grinding halt in the meantime. If you've been treated for Lyme disease and you still have lingering symptoms that are affecting your quality of life, see your doctor to discuss other treatment options. In some cases, treating chronic Lyme disease in ways that are similar to approaches for fibromyalgia or chronic fatigue syndrome can make a difference.

By itself, being exhausted doesn't mean you have an infection. But if you also have symptoms—even vague or subtle ones such as muscle aches, joint pain, a lingering sore throat, nausea, or other unexplained changes that could suggest a bacterial or viral infection—it's important to get these checked out by your doctor. In many cases, blood tests can easily determine if you have an infection. If you do, the sooner you have it treated, the better your chances are of putting an end to your fatigue (and other unpleasant symptoms) and preventing long-term complications.

CHAPTER TWELVE

The Energy Drain of Pain

IT'S HARD TO BELIEVE that things are right with the world when you're in considerable pain. After all, when you hurt, you aren't comfortable in your body, you don't feel like yourself, and you may find it harder to focus because the pain is distracting, if not downright consuming. So it's not surprising that ongoing or chronic pain can drain your energy, leaving you feeling like a pale, diminished version of yourself. The latest research illustrates the breadth of these effects: In a 2014 study involving 5,906 people, researchers at the University of Iceland found that women who had chronic back pain, neck discomfort, or fibromyalgia were twice as likely to report lower satisfaction with life and higher levels of stress and depressive symptoms, and nearly three times more likely to report sleep disturbances, as their pain-free counterparts. In a 2014 study, researchers from Harvard Medical School and Brigham and Women's Hospital in Boston found that 47 percent of people with rheumatoid arthritis reported moderate to high levels of pain and fatigue even with low levels of inflammation. Three out of four people with chronic widespread muscle pain report having fatigue, and as many as 94 percent of people with chronic fatigue syndrome—the vast majority of whom are women—report muscle pain.

The reality is, muscle pain and fatigue may not be independent conditions; they share a common biochemical pathway that is disrupted in chronic pain conditions. Chronic pain may be characterized by abnormalities in brain chemicals such as serotonin and norepinephrine, which can lead to low energy, mood changes, and impaired mental and physical performance. The pain often worsens as neurochemical changes in your body increase your sensitivity to pain, which makes you feel pain in other parts of your body that don't normally hurt. It's a vicious cycle.

What's more, research has found a bona fide connection for what many people have discovered through personal experience—that ongoing or chronic pain can lead to depression, which in turn leads to fatigue ranging from mild to debilitating (thus triggering that vicious cycle). In fact, a 2009 study from researchers at Wayne State University in Detroit found that 35 percent of people with chronic pain also suffer from major depression. And a 2014 study from the Netherlands found that people who had a history of depression were more likely to have a recurrence of depression if they developed ongoing pain (or an increase in the number of pain locations or pain severity) than people who developed a chronic disease. Whether chronic pain or depression causes the other condition or they simply coexist isn't entirely understood, but this much has been ascertained: Chronic pain and depression ride on the same circuitry in the central nervous system. The neurochemicals norepinephrine and serotonin play a central role in the pain-fighting pathway in the brain—and they're involved in depression as well. Plus, some areas of the brain that regulate pain are also involved in the processing of emotions and the regulation of moods. As a result, experiencing chronic pain can trigger changes in these brain regions and neurotransmitter levels, and these shifts can knock you off balance emotionally or alter your thinking abilities, leaving you feeling foggy and fatigued.

In addition to these common links among pain, depression, and fatigue, different forms of chronic pain lead to exhaustion in other ways. What follows is a look at what these are and what steps to take if you suspect you have one of these conditions.

FIBROMYALGIA

A disorder that's characterized by widespread musculoskeletal pain and fatigue, as well as reduced cognitive function, fibromyalgia is often misdiagnosed and misunderstood, even though it's the second most common musculoskeletal condition (after osteoarthritis). More than 12 million people in the United States, most of whom are women between the ages of 25 and 60, have fibromyalgia. In fact, women are 10 times more likely to develop this disorder than men, but no one knows what's behind the gender gap.

Fibromyalgia features a varied array of symptoms, but nearly all people with the condition experience widespread pain, incapacitating fatigue, anxiety, or depression. The pain is often described as muscles that feel like they've been overworked or overstretched—but without exercise. Burning, twitching, or stabbing pain in the muscles is common; specific tender points on the body that are painful to the touch are a critical part of diagnosing the disease. Some researchers theorize that people with fibromyalgia have a gene or genes that cause them to react intensely to stimuli that most people would not perceive as painful. Fibromyalgia is thought to magnify normal pain sensations by altering the way the brain and spinal cord process pain signals, which leads to a heightened sensitivity to touch and discomfort. It has repeatedly been found that patients who suffer from this condition have elevated levels of a neurotransmitter called substance P, which is involved in transmitting pain impulses to and from the brain and spinal cord.

Joint pain in the shoulders and hips is common, and this is often mistaken for osteoarthritis, bursitis, or tendinitis. However, the pain of these conditions is localized to a specific area, whereas the pain and stiffness associated with fibromyalgia are more widespread. Many fibromyalgia sufferers also have headaches; temporomandibular joint disorders; irritable bowel syndrome, or incontinence; dryness in the mouth, nose, and eyes; hypersensitivity to cold and/or heat; trouble concentrating (often called fibro fog); and numbness or tingling in the fingers and/or feet.

While the underlying cause of fibromyalgia isn't known, there are several theories, and most researchers now believe that fibromyalgia results not from a single event but from a combination of many physical and emotional factors. Sometimes symptoms of fibromyalgia begin after a physical trauma or surgery, an infection, or a significant form of psychological stress. In other people, there isn't a single event that triggers the onset; instead, the symptoms gradually set in and add up over time. Some researchers theorize that poor physical conditioning plays a role in the development of fibromyalgia; another theory suggests that "microtrauma" (very slight injury, often brought on by repetitive overuse) to muscles may lead to an ongoing cycle of pain and fatigue with fibromyalgia.

In any case, people who get fibromyalgia are believed to have a biological vulnerability to it that may stem in part from a genetic component. Those who have a close family member with the disorder are more likely to develop it themselves. In addition, people with fibromyalgia appear to have low levels of serotonin and norepinephrine, and the regulation of dopamine seems to be flawed in fibromyalgia sufferers. The net effect of these neurotransmitter abnormalities is a lower threshold for feeling and tolerating pain. (Abnormalities in some of these same neurotransmitters are also linked with depression and anxiety.) It isn't known if these neurotransmitter abnormalities stem from a genetic disorder or come with the onset of the disease.

Meanwhile, emotional stress may be a trigger for the development of fibromyalgia in those who are already at risk for biological reasons. In a 2013 study involving patients at eight study centers, researchers in Germany examined the link between fibromyalgia and post-traumatic stress disorder (PTSD) and found that in 67 percent of people with both conditions, their most extreme traumatic experience and subsequent PTSD symptoms preceded the onset of their chronic widespread pain. A 2009 study from Israel found that fibromyalgia was highly prevalent 3 years later among people who suffered physical injury and extreme stress from a major train crash.

Adding insult to misery, many people with fibromyalgia experience insomnia, disordered sleep, or nonrestorative sleep (meaning that it's light, fragmented, and unrefreshing). In an unfortunate cascade effect, disordered sleep may lead to lower levels of the neurotransmitter serotonin, which increases pain sensitivity. This higher pain sensitivity leads to more sleep problems and more fatigue, which may trigger anxiety about the problem. It's a detrimental loop.

Fibromyalgia is a tricky disorder to diagnose, in part because there is no blood test to definitively confirm its presence (though blood tests are often ordered to exclude other possibilities). There is, however, a blood test called FM/a that purportedly measures proteins in the blood that lessen pain (people with fibromyalgia can't produce normal quantities of these proteins). Yet many experts don't rely on this test because it's still new and not every fibromyalgia patient will have a positive result. In the meantime, other tests for the condition

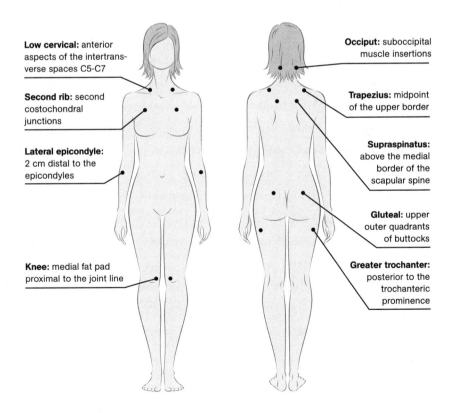

Low cervical: anterior aspects of the intertransverse spaces C5-C7

Second rib: second costochondral junctions

Lateral epicondyle: 2 cm distal to the epicondyles

Knee: medial fat pad proximal to the joint line

Occiput: suboccipital muscle insertions

Trapezius: midpoint of the upper border

Supraspinatus: above the medial border of the scapular spine

Gluteal: upper outer quadrants of buttocks

Greater trochanter: posterior to the trochanteric prominence are in development. The traditional mode of diagnosis is for a physician to check 18 specific points on a person's body to see which of them are tender and painful when pressed firmly; in the past, if 11 out of the 18 points were tender, the person was diagnosed with fibromyalgia. More recently, a consensus has developed that allows a diagnosis to be made if someone has experienced widespread pain in all four quadrants of the body for at least 3 months.

A few years ago, Mary Beth, a 34-year-old single woman who works as a receptionist in a dentist's office, came to see me after going from one doctor to another, seeking relief for her extreme fatigue, migraines, and aching pain in her shoulders and hips (pain that happened to get worse with exercise). She had a long history of irritable bowel syndrome, with waxing and waning symptoms, and she had recently been diagnosed with depression and generalized anxiety disorder. She was put on Prozac, which she discontinued because she found it too sedating. Mary Beth arrived with an 18-inch-high stack of papers—her medical history and records from previous doctors—in a legal file box; they had been carefully organized by date, year, type of specialist, working diagnosis, and treatment/referrals recommended. At the time, she had taken an unpaid leave of absence from work to "try to get to the bottom" of her illness; the previous year, she had used 6 months of paid medical leave for the same purpose but did not find relief.

Mary Beth also complained of mental fogginess and an inability to concentrate, as well as dry skin, hair, mouth, and eyes. She appeared extremely anxious and spoke quickly but lost her train of thought easily. During the physical exam, 11 out of 18 of her tender points were positive for pain, so I referred her to a rheumatology medical group that specializes in fibromyalgia—and she was indeed diagnosed with the disorder as well as depression (again). She was treated with an antiseizure drug called Lyrica (pregabalin), and she started a graded exercise program. Six months later, her pain was 90 percent better, and her fatigue had improved by 30 percent—a relative success story.

There is no cure for fibromyalgia, nor is there a treatment that will address all of the symptoms associated with the disorder. Approaches usually

include a combination of medications, exercises, and behavioral techniques. On the medication front, Lyrica is often prescribed for fibromyalgia pain, as are serotonin and norepinephrine reuptake inhibitors (SNRIs) like Cymbalta (duloxetine), Savella (milnacipran), and Effexor (venlafaxine). Low doses of older tricyclic antidepressants (such as amitriptyline) have been found to be effective in treating fibromyalgia pain, as has a narcotic-like pain-reliever called Ultram (tramadol). Muscle relaxants like Flexeril (cyclobenzaprine) can provide pain relief, but they can also be sedating and habit forming, so they're best used with caution.

Alternative therapies such as massage, acupuncture, chiropractic manipulation, and myofascial release (a soft-tissue therapy that involves applying gentle, sustained pressure into the myofascial connective tissue to eliminate pain and improve range of motion) have been shown to help with pain control. Interestingly, a 2013 study published in the *Journal of Bodywork and Movement Therapies* found that myofascial release was particularly effective at producing consistent reductions in pain in the neck and upper back among people with fibromyalgia. In addition, deep breathing techniques, hypnosis, and maintaining a regular sleep schedule also mitigate fibromyalgia fatigue. The American Pain Society recommends moderately intense aerobic exercise at least two or three times per week. In a 2014 study involving 199 adults with fibromyalgia, researchers from Indiana University–Purdue University Indianapolis found that participants who increased their steps per day experienced greater improvements in physical function, pain-related interference with activities, and depressive symptoms; every increase of 1,000 steps per day yielded noteworthy improvements.

MIGRAINES

There's a close link between fatigue and migraines, which are classically one-sided, throbbing headaches that may be accompanied by nausea, vomiting, and sensitivity to light. Before, during, and after a migraine attack, many migraine sufferers—as much as 84 percent, according to some studies—report an overall lack of energy. Further, a 2002 study from Brazil found that 67 percent of the participating migraine sufferers met the criteria for chronic fatigue syndrome. In some cases, the fatigue is so severe and disabling that it's considered a syndrome in its own right, one that's called migraine fatigue; the pain is significant enough to interfere with a person's ability to perform daily activities and compromise her overall quality of life. But there's even more to the migraine-fatigue connection. Fatigue and too little sleep can not only trigger painful migraines but also cause additional migraine symptoms such as vertigo. What's more, fatigue is often associated with depression in people who suffer from migraines.

Approximately 28 million people in the United States suffer from migraines, and these killer headaches are more common among women than men. Among women who get migraines, 25 percent suffer four or more per month, and each migraine can last from 4 hours to 3 days. There's a hereditary component to migraines: Eighty percent of migraine sufferers have a family history of these debilitating headaches. If one parent has migraines, his or her child has a 50 percent chance of developing them; if both parents have a history of migraines, the risk jumps to 75 percent.

To this day, the exact causes of migraines are poorly understood, though they are believed to involve changes in the brain. Among them: hyperactive nerve cells that send signals to the blood vessels, causing them to constrict and then dilate, thereby triggering painful sensations; activation of the trigeminal nerve, which evokes a series of events in the meninges (layers of connective tissue covering the brain and spinal cord) and the brain stem, events that lead to pain; and changes in brain chemicals such as serotonin and inflammatory substances. People with migraines may inherit the tendency to be affected by certain triggers such as sleep loss, bright lights, monthly hormonal fluctuations, barometric pressure changes, emotional stress, certain compounds in foods, and changes in sleep patterns.

Once you develop a tendency toward migraines, there's no way to reverse that vulnerability, but there are ways to manage these debilitating headaches. A variety of medications—including nonsteroidal anti-inflammatory drugs (NSAIDs), acetaminophen-aspirin-caffeine combinations (like Excedrin, which has all three ingredients, or Anacin, which contains only aspirin and caffeine), triptans (such as Imitrex/sumatriptan), and antinausea drugs—are used to treat migraines and stop the symptoms after they've begun. In addition, alternative techniques such as biofeedback and transcranial magnetic stimulation devices may short-circuit migraines after they start.

For those who have four or more debilitating migraine attacks per month, preventive medications—such as beta-blockers, calcium channel blockers, tricyclic antidepressants, antiseizure drugs, and Botox injections—may be recommended. When taken daily, preventive medications have been found to reduce the frequency, severity, and duration of migraines, and they may enhance the effectiveness of symptom-relieving drugs that are used during an acute attack. It's also important for all sufferers to try to identify their personal migraine triggers and avoid them as much as possible.

Last year, Donna, a 45-year-old teacher and mother of one, came to see me because she was experiencing overwhelming fatigue. It was so severe that she would come home from work at 3:30 p.m. and crawl into bed for the night. She also had migraines two or three times a week, with nausea, vomiting, light sensitivity, and occasionally vision problems in one eye. Donna believed the fatigue was triggering her headaches, because after she slept for 17 hours, the pain would go away, but she'd have intense residual fatigue the following day, which would spark the migraine cycle again. At the time, she was taking large quantities of NSAIDs and over-the-counter sleep aids (like Nyquil and Unisom) to treat the pain. Her blood work showed slightly elevated creatinine, a marker of early kidney damage from excessive use of NSAIDs. I referred her to a neurologist, and together we convinced her to try propranolol, a beta-blocker that prevents migraines when it's taken on a daily basis. During the following 2 months, she experienced only one migraine per month, and her fatigue dropped dramatically.

ARTHRITIS

Pain is arguably the most common and troublesome symptom of arthritis, but fatigue runs a close second. Rheumatoid arthritis (RA), an autoimmune disorder, is directly linked to fatigue through the pathophysiology of the disease; in fact, fatigue can precede the onset of other symptoms by weeks or months. But even with osteoarthritis (OA), which stems from age-related wear and tear on the joints, dealing with pain on a day-to-day basis wears you down and causes fatigue. Being fatigued, in turn, can worsen the pain of arthritis and make the condition more difficult to manage.

There are several ways in which arthritis causes fatigue. For starters, with both RA and OA, inflammatory cytokines (proteins in the blood) are released, and these substances trigger fatigue. In addition, many of the medications that are used to treat OA and RA—such as narcotic analgesics, some prescription NSAIDs, antidepressants, blood pressure medications, and sleep aids—are considered energy zappers; then, too, corticosteroids, which fight inflammation, may cause daytime lethargy by interfering with sleep at night. Anemia is fairly common with arthritis, particularly RA, whether it's because of the disease process itself, an ulcer induced by frequent use of NSAIDs, or even the effect of inflammatory cytokines on the body's ability to make red blood cells. Not surprisingly, one of the primary symptoms of anemia, which is related to poor circulation of oxygen in the blood, is fatigue.

Plus, if the pain of arthritis makes it difficult to fall asleep or wakes you during the night, you can end up wiped out the next day. Indeed, sleep difficulties are often what motivate people with arthritis to seek medical care. Because the pain of RA or OA can make it difficult to perform normal daily activities, it's hardly surprising that depression often goes hand in hand with the disease; depression also may stem from fluctuations in hormones and neurotransmitters that are related to the stress of having a chronic health condition. Whatever the underlying reason may be, a 2014 study from Taiwan found that people with RA were more than twice as likely to develop a depressive disorder over a 10-year follow-up period as their peers who didn't have RA.

Dozens of different medications are used to treat arthritis, including pain relievers (primarily over-the-counter analgesics and prescription opioid analgesics), anti-inflammatory drugs (from oral NSAIDs to topical treatments), disease-modifying drugs (DMARDs, which stop or slow the disease's progression), biologics (genetically engineered medications that control the immune response), and corticosteroids (to treat inflammation in the joints). In addition, some supplements such as ASU (short for avocado-soybean unsaponifiables, a natural vegetable extract made from avocado and soybean oils) and omega-3 fatty acids (such as fish oil capsules) have been found to improve symptoms. Moreover, some alternative remedies—such as acupuncture, massage, and meditation—may ease the pain significantly. It's also important to stay active with regular physical activity (walking, swimming, and yoga are easy on the joints) and to lose weight if you're overweight (to lessen pressure on the joints).

A couple of years ago, Kate, a married mother of two, came to me complaining of having 3 weeks of severe fatigue, intermittent fevers, intolerance to cold, and an almost daily headache. A physical exam didn't reveal anything abnormal, so I sent her blood work to the lab and we scheduled a follow-up appointment for 3 weeks later. Two weeks later, Kate called from the ER, where she had gone after she woke up with pain and stiffness at the base of her left hand and wrist. Her sister has multiple sclerosis (MS), so Kate thought she might be experiencing the initial signs of MS; her sister's first symptoms were weakness and tingling in the lower legs. The ER doctor suspected Kate might have Lyme disease, but blood tests revealed that she didn't—she had rheumatoid arthritis. She was put on a DMARD, her fatigue subsided completely, and her joint symptoms are now well controlled.

TEMPOROMANDIBULAR JOINT DISORDERS

Sometimes these disorders are erroneously referred to as TMJ (which stands for the temporomandibular joint), but the correct acronym is TMD. Temporomandibular joint disorders, which are more common among women than men, are a group of conditions involving the jaw, the jaw joint, and surrounding facial muscles that control chewing and movement of the jaw. Fatigue is a frequent complaint with jaw-joint dysfunction, as is pain or tenderness in the face, the jaw joint area, the neck and shoulders, and in or around the ear when you chew, speak, or open your mouth wide. Some people with TMD are unable to open their mouths fully, or they struggle with having their jaws get "stuck" or "locked" in the open- or closed-mouth position. Clicking, popping, or grating sounds in the jaw joint are also common when chewing or opening or closing the mouth. Occasionally, swelling occurs on one or both sides of the face.

As for the fatigue factor, this is how it happens: For one thing, jaw pain can disrupt sleep. In addition, some research suggests that dysfunction of the trigeminal nerve (the nerve that extends to the jaw muscles that are used for chewing) is a more direct cause of fatigue, because it can stimulate the fatigue centers located in the brain stem. Some researchers also theorize that since the trigeminal nerve communicates with the brain's limbic system, which affects our emotions, memories, and mental and physical arousal, pain in the nerve also may drain our energy levels.

Whatever the underlying physiologic mechanism is, TMD has numerous causes, including direct injury (such as being punched in the face or injured in a car accident), grinding or clenching of the teeth (which puts a lot of pressure on the temporomandibular joint), arthritis in the TMJ, or stress (which can cause you to tighten your facial and jaw muscles or clench your teeth). The condition is usually diagnosed during a physical exam, but occasionally an MRI or a CT scan is recommended to investigate the extent of the damage and dysfunction. Treatment for TMD includes a mouth guard that's worn at night to prevent grinding, NSAIDs (to reduce pain and swelling), transcutaneous electric nerve stimulation, and trigger point injections into the facial muscles (to provide pain relief). Surgery is a last resort for the most severe cases.

CHRONIC BACK, NECK, AND SHOULDER PAIN

The human back is a complex structure that comprises interconnecting nerves, muscles, bones, ligaments, tendons, disks, and the spinal cord. The most common cause of back pain is muscle strain, but any ongoing problem in the back—whether it's from a muscle sprain, a slipped disk, arthritis, or degenerating bones and disks—can cause pain and fatigue. Specifically, the pain may trigger muscle spasms that overwhelm the nervous system, resulting in substantial fatigue throughout the body.

Back pain is one of the most common health complaints in the United States—8 out of 10 people will have it at some point, according to the National Institutes of Health—and it's especially common among those between the ages of 40 and 80. While both men and women can develop back pain at any time, women are particularly vulnerable during pregnancy (partly because of the extra body weight they're carrying but also because pregnancy hormones relax the joints and ligaments), when toting heavy purses or bags (which can result in an overuse injury and misalignment of the shoulders, neck, or back), or if they are well endowed (having large breasts can alter a woman's posture and put pressure directly on the upper back).

When the pain becomes chronic (meaning it lasts longer than 3 months) or it's severe, the first step is to see your doctor to figure out what's causing the aching or throbbing sensations. (This is true whether the pain is in your neck, your upper back, or your lower back.) Once the source of the problem has been unmasked by x-rays, MRI, or CT scans, treatment may involve the use of over-the-counter pain relievers to ease discomfort and anti-inflammatory drugs to reduce inflammation, the application of hot or cold packs or topical analgesics, exercise (which may be the last thing you feel like doing, but it actually speeds recovery), steroid or analgesic injections, and/or complementary approaches (such as acupuncture or manipulation). Most people with chronic back pain don't need surgery; it's usually reserved for cases in which other treatments don't produce sufficient pain relief or improvement in functionality.

So that's the story on how and why pain can drain your energy, not to mention severely compromise the quality of your life and state of mind. If you're suffering from ongoing pain of any kind along with fatigue, note them on the symptom checklist (found in Chapter 14) and schedule a visit to your doctor sooner, not later; it's a mistake to try to tough it out. There are good treatments for many forms of chronic pain—and many more are in the pipeline—so there's no reason to suffer. Moreover, working with your doctor to get to the bottom of your symptoms can help you manage the underlying condition and prevent complications. In the process of repairing the drain of pain, you can regain at least some of your get-up-and-go and begin to feel like yourself again.

CHAPTER THIRTEEN

An Exhausted Mind: Depression, Dysthymia, and Anxiety

MANY PEOPLE THINK THAT depression equals sadness. Sometimes that's true, but it doesn't have to be. For some people, fatigue, malaise, apathy, and a loss of interest in normally enjoyable activities are more common symptoms of depression than feeling blue or having crying jags. Even among those who do feel sad or downbeat, fatigue can be an accompanying symptom of major depression or dysthymia (a milder, chronic form of depression). After monitoring 3,201 people from 15 primary-care centers in 14 countries for a year, researchers from Greece found that people who were depressed were four times more likely to develop fatigue, while those who had unexplained fatigue were nearly three times more likely to become depressed. Their conclusion: "Unexplained fatigue and depression might act as independent risk factors for each other." That's why depression is one of the most important things to look for when searching for the cause of unexplained fatigue.

While a large body of research has established a close link between depression and fatigue, exactly how they interact is not yet completely understood. Part of this could be because depression and fatigue feed off each other in a vicious cycle that makes it hard to determine where one begins and the other ends. In many ways, they have different risk factors, but there are some overlaps. For example, regular physical activity is known to help protect against depression, and it has also been suggested that physical deconditioning may be an important factor in the development of unexplained fatigue. Sleep is another critical part of the equation: Depression often disrupts sleep patterns, which can leave you feeling unrefreshed or even wiped out the next day. This sleep loss aggravates the symptoms of depression, leading to an ongoing cycle of insomnia (or interrupted sleep), followed by fatigue and an exacerbation of depression symptoms.

In another powerful mind–body effect, fatigue has a negative effect on brain chemistry over time. Researchers have found a significant drop in activity in the frontal lobes of the brain in excessively tired people. What's more, frontal lobe dysfunction is thought to play a role in the mood and behavior changes that accompany depression.

Fatigue can also be a lingering symptom of depression. In a 2014 review of the published literature on the subject, researchers from Massachusetts General Hospital and Harvard Medical School found that "fatigue is highly prevalent as a residual symptom" of major depressive disorder (MDD)—and it's "not being adequately addressed by standard antidepressant therapies." In a 2010 study from Greece, more than 90 percent of patients with MDD had severe fatigue despite the fact that more than 80 percent of them were already taking antidepressant medications. Not only is depression-related fatigue slow to respond to treatment with antidepressants, but the Harvard researchers say the presence of residual fatigue predicts that someone recovering from MDD is more likely to have a relapse. It also forecasts a greater likelihood that she'll experience impairments in her ability to function psychologically and socially.

Depression has two sets of symptoms that can rise and fall relatively independently of each other. One set consists of distress-related symptoms such as depressed mood, worry, negative thinking, and dread; the other set affects energy level, motivation, and a person's ability to enjoy activities or experiences. Some treatments for depression (including many antidepressants) tend to be more effective for the distress symptoms than they are for fatigue and lack of energy. In fact, while antidepressants improve symptoms of sadness, worry, and negativity, they can trigger an unmotivated, tired state in the process.

If anyone knows this, it's Ashley, a 28-year-old law school student with a strong family history of depression. She had been diagnosed with the disorder through student health services at her school 6 months before our visit. At the time of her diagnosis, she reported that she "felt sad" and had a despondent, irritable mood for most of the day. She also experienced fatigue (yet had difficulty sleeping), loss of interest in activities that usually brought her pleasure, concentration problems (with a resulting change in her school performance), weight gain, and recurring thoughts of death (but not suicide). During this period, she spent most of her day in bed. Her psychiatrist had been treating her with weekly therapy sessions and a selective serotonin reuptake inhibitor (SSRI). Ashley came to see me because while her symptoms of depression had lifted dramatically, she felt more fatigued than ever.

Even though her mental motivation to "get back to life" was restored, physically her energy was so depleted that she still spent hours upon hours in bed. She suspected something medical was underlying her situation. But since her examination and blood work didn't show anything abnormal, I suggested reconsidering her antidepressant medication. While she was hesitant to change a regimen she felt was working overall, in collaboration with her psychiatrist we started her on a less-sedating SSRI, which improved her energy level by about 60 percent within 6 weeks. She regained enough get-up-and-go to hit the gym, which improved her exhaustion as well. Two years later, she was depression-free and off meds (she continued with psychotherapy)—and her energy was back to normal.

Major depression itself can cause a state of lethargy or lack of energy that's called anergia. This chronic state of low energy is associated with mental, emotional, and physical fatigue that's difficult to treat. The physical symptoms include reduced activity, tiredness, decreased physical endurance, general weakness, slowness or sluggishness, nonrestorative sleep, and

A Common Case of Mistaken Identity

Chronic fatigue syndrome (CFS) is often initially diagnosed as depression, which isn't surprising since it shares many of the symptoms of depression and the two disorders often coexist. In a 2008 study of patients with chronic fatigue syndrome, researchers from the University of Toronto found that 36 percent also suffered from depression and lower levels of mastery and self-esteem. The incidence of depression was higher among female patients, as well as among those from a lower income bracket and those for whom pain limited their physical activity. This type of research draws attention to the fact that the medical community should be aware of the need to look for and treat both conditions simultaneously.

sleepiness. The cognitive symptoms include impaired concentration, attention, and mental endurance, as well as slowed thinking. The emotional symptoms include decreased motivation or apathy, an aversion to making an effort to do things, lessened interest in normally interesting activities, feeling overwhelmed and unable to cope, and feeling down or low.

If it's left untreated, persistent fatigue can even contribute to a longer, more severe bout of depression, research suggests. Fatigue itself is also one of the main causes of disability in depression, and it makes it harder for people to take the necessary steps to get effective treatment.

WHAT'S IN A NAME?

It's important to distinguish between major depression and milder forms. Major depressive disorder (MDD) is characterized by having a depressed mood most of the day and a loss of interest in one's usual activities and relationships—

symptoms that are present every day for at least 2 weeks. Other symptoms of MDD might include fatigue or loss of energy nearly every day; feelings of worthlessness or guilt; impaired concentration or indecisiveness; insomnia or hypersomnia (excessive sleeping) almost every day; a markedly diminished interest in or enjoyment of normally enjoyable activities (a symptom called anhedonia); restlessness or feeling slowed down; recurring thoughts of death or suicide; and/or significant weight loss or gain (a change of more than 5 percent in body weight in a month).

Dysthymia, by contrast, is a chronic but milder form of depression that lasts for at least 2 years. It's a steady state of feeling down, but it's less debilitating than MDD. (Eeyore, from *Winnie-the-Pooh,* is one of the best examples of a character with dysthymia that I can think of from popular culture.) The primary symptom is a low, dark, or sad mood on most days of the week. Other symptoms can include low energy or fatigue, feelings of hopelessness, sleeping too much or too little, low self-esteem, concentration problems, a loss of appetite, or a pattern of overeating.

Approximately 10 percent of adults in the United States currently have some form of depression, according to the Centers for Disease Control and Prevention, and up to 25 percent of adults will suffer an episode of major depression at some point in their lifetimes, according to the National Institute of Mental Health. Women are twice as susceptible to depression as men, and there are numerous theories as to why. These include hormonal fluctuations (during the menstrual cycle, pregnancy, perimenopause, and menopause), genetic influences, and work overload (from juggling career and home responsibilities). Another theory is that women's thinking styles— namely, the tendency to ruminate about problems—may be a factor as well, whether this habit comes naturally or is learned.

Depression tends to be more prevalent among adults between the ages of 45 and 64 and among those who have a family history of the disorder. If a member of your immediate family (a parent or sibling) has suffered from depression, your risk of developing it is three times higher than it is for someone who doesn't have a family history of the disorder, according to research from Virginia Commonwealth University.

While I have a strong family history of depression, in my case I think my fatigue triggered the major depressive episode I experienced during medical school: Exhaustion was my overwhelming symptom. I had severe fatigue and low motivation. It was hard to wake up in the morning, and getting through a standard 8-to-5 day was way too much for me. The only thing that seemed appealing was going to sleep, and as a result, I wasn't enjoying or able to do things I usually looked forward to. My first-year advisor suggested I see a psychiatrist, who diagnosed me with major depression. Psychotherapy was helpful, as were some antidepressants. One in particular, Wellbutrin (bupropion), was mildly stimulating, and it perked me up by about 10 percent. But because my exhaustion was still unbearable despite the improvement in my mood and motivation, I embarked on my journey to find the underlying causes of my fatigue, and I later discovered that chronic fatigue syndrome was at the root of it.

Common triggers for major depression include grief (from losing a loved one through death, divorce, or separation); social isolation or loneliness; major life transitions such as moving, graduating from school, changing jobs, or retiring; personal conflicts in relationships (whether it's with a significant other, a boss, or a close friend); and physical, sexual, or emotional abuse.

Depression is diagnosed based on a screening test (such as the Beck Depression Inventory) that assesses your personal symptoms and behavior patterns, after your doctor has ruled out other potential medical causes. Making the diagnosis may seem like a no-brainer, but it isn't always, because depression can manifest in so many different ways. One woman may be obviously sad and blue, another may seem irritable and agitated, while yet another may present with apathy and low energy. As with fatigue, it's common for women to explain away symptoms that may suggest depression, blaming them on stress overload, too little sleep, or something else. Meanwhile, other studies have revealed that exhausted women are more likely than men are to describe themselves as "depressed," though they may not actually meet the criteria for clinical depression.

A few years ago, Nora, a 34-year-old nanny who takes care of a close friend's young daughter, seemed to go through a personality transformation. Over the course of 8 months, she went from being pleasant, punctual, and upbeat to more subdued and less reliable; she was frequently late or absent. She also became less active with the child and said this was because she was constantly tired. One day when my friend got home from work, she found the nanny asleep on the couch in front of *Oprah* while her then 2-year-old daughter was toddling around the kitchen unsupervised. That's when my friend sent Nora to see me.

Nora described relentless exhaustion, to the point where she could barely keep her eyes open. She was having trouble falling asleep at night and waking up in the morning, and she admitted to sneaking frequent naps while on the job. But she didn't describe a "depressed mood" and said she had "nothing to be sad about." Two years earlier, she had left her family and children in the Philippines to work in the United States, but since she felt that was the right thing to do, she insisted she didn't experience sadness or a sense of loss about it. She didn't have weight or appetite disturbances, changes in her relationships or moods, difficulty concentrating, or any thoughts of death— she was just bone-tired. Because her physical exam was within normal limits, I suggested she talk to a therapist; Nora initially refused, but a few weeks later she agreed when her fatigue and lethargy worsened. She was diagnosed with major depressive disorder and treated with psychotherapy and antidepressants; within a couple of months, her fatigue resolved completely.

It's important to get depression diagnosed properly and treated effectively; otherwise, it can have a long-lasting effect on your mental and physical health as well as your energy. Antidepressant medications are often the first line of treatment used for clinical depression, and they are prescribed alone or in addition to psychotherapy (usually cognitive behavioral therapy or interpersonal therapy). By increasing the availability of neurotransmitters—

including serotonin, norepinephrine, and dopamine—or by changing the sensitivity of the receptors for these chemical messengers, antidepressants improve mood. Because there are so many different kinds of antidepressants—selective serotonin reuptake inhibitors (SSRIs), serotonin and norepinephrine reuptake inhibitors (SNRIs), and tricyclic antidepressants, to name the most common ones—finding the one that works for you may take some time and a bit of trial and error. But don't let that discourage you: Six out of 10 people will begin to feel better with the first antidepressant they are prescribed, according to the US Department of Health and Human Services, but it often takes at least 6 weeks to experience the full benefits of the drugs.

When medications provide initial relief from symptoms of depression, many people experience an energy boost that allows them to take a more active part in their recovery. This might include psychotherapy in the form of cognitive behavioral therapy, which focuses on how your thoughts and behaviors contribute to your depression and other feelings, or interpersonal therapy, which focuses on how your relationships may play a role in your depression. To date, the most effective treatment for depression is a combination of antidepressants and psychotherapy—each is more powerful together than either is alone.

In addition, it's important to modify your lifestyle habits to support your mood-management efforts. This includes practicing good, consistent sleep habits (see Chapter 3) and exercising regularly (see Chapter 6), which can improve your mood and promote better sleep. In fact, research from Duke University found that regular exercise relieves depression as well as antidepressants do and keeps it in remission after a year. What's more, a single 30-minute session of aerobic exercise enhances feelings of energy and decreases fatigue, according to a 2013 study from the University of Georgia.

Sticking with a healthy diet (see Chapter 5) also recharges you. Consuming foods higher in fat and sugar increases daytime sleepiness and/or energy crashes, whereas a diet higher in complex carbohydrates (such as whole grains, fruits, and vegetables) and lean proteins (such as skinless poultry, fish, seafood, eggs, beans, and legumes) boosts alertness and daytime energy. Eating plenty of omega-3 fatty acids, found in cold-water fish, flaxseeds, walnuts, and other foods, may help relieve depression, too, according to some studies. You should remember to drink plenty of water throughout the day, and avoid alcohol if you're depressed.

Meanwhile, there are a variety of alternative therapies for depression—including meditation, acupuncture, hypnosis, yoga, herbal remedies (such as St. John's wort and SAMe, which is short for S-adenosylmethionine, a chemical found naturally in the body that is involved in a variety of body functions), and others—that have yielded mixed results in research settings, although some people swear by them. In a 2004 study published in the *Journal of Affective Disorders*, 61 pregnant women with major depression were treated with acupuncture specifically tailored for depression, general acupuncture, or massage therapy. After 8 weeks, 69 percent of those who were treated with acupuncture that specifically targeted depression no longer met the full criteria for MDD, and they had at least a 50 percent reduction in their depressive symptoms; by comparison, the response rates were lower for those who received general acupuncture or massage therapy. Meanwhile, a 2010 study from Brazil found that people who learned and practiced meditation for an hour a week had a significant reduction in their depression scores and an increased attention span after 5 weeks. And a 2009 study from Japan showed that doing a mindfulness-based meditation program for just 2 weeks reduced depression and anxiety among patients being treated for cancer.

Fortunately, with various forms of treatment, two-thirds of people with major depression recover, although there are people for whom it's more difficult to find sufficient relief. The good news is, for those who have "treatment-resistant depression"—meaning they've tried several different antidepressants, psychotherapy, or other treatments but still don't feel better—there's a growing arsenal of weapons against the tenacious mood disorder. New, stronger medications—such as Brintellix (vortioxetine), Fetzima (levomilnacipran), and Symbyax (fluoxetine and olanzapine)—have become available, and emerging

(continued on page 191)

Breaking Bad Emotional Habits

Believe it or not, a variety of patterns that occur inside your mind can deplete your energy and/or increase your risk of becoming depressed or anxious. I'm not just talking about the superwoman syndrome, whereby some women feel like they have to take care of everything and everyone themselves and push themselves to go above and beyond the call of duty. There are also other sneaky and insidious emotional habits that damage your well-being and vitality—and women are especially vulnerable due to our work-family juggling acts and our natural thinking patterns.

Fortunately, you can learn to come to your own emotional rescue. The first step is to identify the habit and then take steps to change it. Here's how:

The Habit: Being a Perfectionist

THE SIGNS AND RISKS: You hold yourself to incredibly high standards and feel as if you've failed if you don't meet them. Overall, you feel as though nothing you do is quite good enough. The trouble is, being a perfectionist is like having a slave driver on your shoulder, one who constantly pushes and criticizes you, thereby draining your vigor. Moreover, a 2014 study from Curtin University in Perth, Australia, found significant associations between certain aspects of perfectionism (such as concern over mistakes and doubts about one's actions) and pathological worry and generalized anxiety disorder (GAD).

THE REMEDY: Strive for excellence, not perfection. Make sure your standards and goals are realistic and attainable. Ask yourself: *Am I holding myself to standards that I would never ask a friend to meet?* Then set priorities and consider what's worth doing your absolute best on and what you can do a "good enough" job on. It helps to focus more on the experience of what you're doing rather than the outcome.

The Habit: Putting Yourself on Guilt Trips

THE SIGNS AND RISKS: You often make yourself feel bad about the choices you've made. You frequently second-guess your actions.

Or you find yourself doing things you don't want to do just to avoid feeling guilty. Unfortunately, putting yourself on frequent guilt trips lowers your self-esteem and/or makes you feel depressed, sapping your energy in the process. What's more, a 2014 study from the University of Illinois at Urbana-Champaign found that a propensity for feeling guilt and shame plays a role in worry and GAD.

THE REMEDY: Question your guilt. When guilty feelings creep in, ask yourself: *Is this a rational, logical thought? What evidence is there to support what I'm saying to myself?* If there's no basis for the guilt, it's likely to dissipate on its own. If there is a basis, consider what your guilt is trying to tell you. If you've done something wrong or out of sync with your values, try to amend the situation by apologizing or changing your behavior.

The Habit: Squelching Your Feelings

THE SIGNS AND RISKS: You tend to go along with other people's ideas, just to ensure that everyone gets along. You keep angry feelings to yourself because you're afraid of stirring up trouble in your relationships at home or work. And you're afraid of how people will view you if you express anger, frustration, or disappointment. This self-silencing habit can leave you feeling powerless, hopeless, and ultimately depressed. It also may put your health at risk: A 2011 study from the United Kingdom found that people with chronic fatigue syndrome and anorexia nervosa had higher levels of maladaptive beliefs about expressing their emotions to others.

THE REMEDY: Get in touch with your feelings and try to unearth buried ones by keeping a journal. Each day, spend a few minutes writing down your thoughts about various aspects of your life, particularly situations that upset you or leave you uneasy. Start telling people how you feel, using gentle statements (such as "I feel . . .") rather than accusatory ones; explain how the facts behind a situation affected you, and then ask for a specific change you want to have happen.

The Habit: Being a People Pleaser

THE SIGNS AND RISKS: You find it hard to turn down requests from others, even when you don't have the time or desire to take them on. You often find yourself seeking praise or approval in work or social settings. And you generally squirm in the face of conflict because you're afraid of how you're going to come across to others. Keep this up and you could lose self-esteem, which increases your risk of becoming depressed and/or exhausted. Indeed, a 2000 study from the College of William and Mary in Williamsburg, Virginia, found that depressed students scored higher on measures of self-criticism and the need to please others.

THE REMEDY: Challenge your motives. Before you agree to do someone a favor that you really don't have time for, ask yourself why you'd be doing it. If your reason is just to avoid disappointing someone else or to gain their favor and it's at your own expense, think twice about saying yes. Also, recognize the benefit you get out of trying to please others—perhaps it helps you feel needed and important—and look for other ways to get those perks.

The Habit: Ruminating about Your Problems

THE SIGNS AND RISKS: You often mull over upsetting events in your mind as you examine all the facets. As you review the same thoughts and ideas in a cyclical way, you end up spinning your mental wheels, which can make you feel overwhelmed by your problems. Indeed, research suggests that rumination leads people to think about situations with increasing negativity, sending you into a downward spiral of depression and anxiety. In a 2014 study, researchers from Belgium found that increases in depressive symptoms over the course of a week could be predicted by how much the study subjects ruminated.

THE REMEDY: Recognize that you're ruminating, then distract yourself when the habit kicks in. Redirect your attention to an absorbing or engaging activity (such as exercise or an enjoyable hobby), then set problem-solving hours for later, when you can come back to the situation with a fresh perspective. When the designated time arrives, brainstorm solutions by writing down what you think the essential issue is and how it needs to be changed, then generate ideas for what you can do to move toward that goal.

high-tech treatments are showing promise. One is transcranial magnetic stimulation, which uses magnetic pulses similar to those used in MRIs to stimulate areas of the brain that are thought to be involved in depression and mood regulation. Another is vagus nerve stimulation, in which a small device like a pacemaker is implanted in the chest; it sends pulses of electricity to the vagus nerve in the neck and into key areas of the brain in an effort to smooth out mood fluctuations. Electroconvulsive therapy (aka "shock" therapy) is still used as a treatment of last resort for severe or life-threatening cases of treatment-resistant depression.

ANXIETY DISORDERS

Anxiety can cause fatigue, though seldom to the extent that depression does. The physical and emotional symptoms of anxiety are draining for a variety of reasons. Your body uses up energy when it's constantly in a red-alert state and ready to swing into action to deal with potential threats. When a real physical threat doesn't come at you and the adrenaline surges ease up, you'll experience a crash that can result in fatigue. Anxiety causes profound muscle tension throughout the day, which tires out your body and leaves you feeling "drained." Add to this the hormonal and neural changes that occur during times of severe stress (namely, the body's fight-or-flight response that stimulates the release of stress hormones, which have ripple effects on a variety of bodily functions), and the results are anxiety overload and exhaustion.

Meanwhile, anxiety leads to mental exhaustion because it's tiresome to focus on fear and worry. Anxiety triggers a host of rapid, stressful thoughts, and your brain—like a muscle—can run out of strength and energy. The anxious mind-set makes it difficult to fall asleep or stay asleep. Insomnia is a common side effect of anxiety, and the sleepless nights will wipe you out even more, setting up a vicious cycle. In addition, sleep loss can boost anticipatory anxiety (feeling anxious when you anticipate doing something that scares or worries you), according to research from the University of California, Berkeley. Moreover, being perpetually tired makes it harder to cope with stressful situations, so the problem builds up until you cannot resolve difficult situations effectively.

With generalized anxiety disorder (GAD), the most common type of anxiety disorder, free-floating nervousness and worry occur, along with feeling restless, keyed up, or on edge; being easily fatigued; having difficulty concentrating; being irritable; and/or experiencing muscle tension or sleep disturbances (having difficulty falling asleep or staying asleep or having restless or simply unsatisfying sleep). To be diagnosed with GAD, the symptoms need to have occurred for more days than not for at least 6 months. The anxiety doesn't relate to the possibility of having a panic attack (though panic attacks can occur in someone with GAD). It's not about being embarrassed or excessively shy in public (as in social anxiety); it's not about having unreasonable thoughts or fears that lead you to engage in repetitive behaviors (as in obsessive-compulsive disorder). With GAD, the anxiety is general, just as the name suggests, but the nervousness, worry, and/or physical symptoms that are associated with it cause significant distress or impairment in your ability to function at work, at home, socially, and in other areas of your life.

Anxiety disorders affect twice as many women as men, and they tend to run in families. It's believed there are both genetic and learned components to anxiety (it's due to nature and nurture, in other words). A history of trauma and social isolation (or a lack of social connections) and certain medical conditions (such as inflammatory bowel disorders) are also associated with an increased risk of these disorders.

Some people with anxiety feel tired throughout the day or as though they can't focus on the business of life. Others feel tired only after they've had an anxiety attack. The patterns vary considerably. Complicating the picture, anxiety and depression are often intertwined: Sometimes they coexist; in other cases, anxiety causes temporary depression (especially after an anxiety attack) or lasting depression. A study from the Columbia University

College of Physicians and Surgeons found that 85 percent of those with major depression were also diagnosed with generalized anxiety disorder. It's a combination that delivers a powerful one-two punch to your energy.

Because they often run together, anxiety and depression are viewed as the fraternal twins of mood disorders. It's a combination that's challenging to manage. When anxiety occurs with depression, the symptoms of both disorders tend to be more severe than when either disorder occurs on its own; what's more, the symptoms of depression take longer to resolve. The link between chronic stress, depression, and anxiety is complex and incredibly powerful: Long-term elevations in stress hormones (primarily cortisol) can lead to physical changes in the structure of the brain—changes that can increase your sensitivity to pain and emotional stressors and even impair your memory.

Not long ago, Kim, a 50-year-old teacher, came to see me because she thought her thyroid was "off." She'd had a total thyroidectomy nearly 20 years earlier after the birth of her only child—she explained that her doctors at the time told her the surgery would cure her constant crying jags, nervousness, and easily triggered temper. Since then, she had been prescribed the drug Synthroid (levothyroxine), a synthetic thyroid hormone, once daily, with recommended follow-up appointments with her physician to make sure the dosing was correct. Yet she confessed that she "hates doctors" and would at times go for years without an exam. Occasionally, too, she would forget to take her thyroid medicine for several days (this is incredibly dangerous because thyroid hormone is critical for normal bodily functions).

Kim decided to see me because for the previous 4 months, she'd been feeling more nervous and jittery than usual. She was in a constant rage with her family and would have twice-daily episodes during which she'd become short of breath, tremulous, clammy, and dizzy, with her heart pounding and her fingers tingling. During these bouts, she said she'd "hear strange things," as though someone were talking to her even if she was alone. She couldn't identify a trigger for these bouts. She was able to make it through her workday, but when she got home, she'd get right in bed, and she'd feel overwhelmingly tired, as though she had taken a sleeping pill.

Much to my surprise, her thyroid hormone levels were within normal limits, and nothing was unusual on her other lab tests. I referred Kim to a psychiatrist, who diagnosed her with generalized anxiety disorder, panic attacks, and depression. She was started on an SSRI antidepressant. Two months later, she reported fewer episodes of anxiety, improved mood and energy, and no more extreme, sedation-like fatigue.

As in Kim's case, your physician or a mental-health professional can diagnose GAD by asking detailed questions about your symptoms and medical history and using psychological questionnaires to assess patterns of feelings and behaviors. A physical exam and blood tests also may be warranted to make sure an underlying medical condition (such as hyperthyroidism) isn't causing your symptoms. The primary treatments for an anxiety disorder are psychotherapy and medication, and often a combination of the two is used. Cognitive behavioral therapy is one of the most effective approaches to GAD because it focuses largely on teaching you specific skills to help you dial down your anxiety and better manage the activities or situations that tend to trigger it. Several types of medications are used for GAD, including antidepressants (such as SSRIs and SNRIs) and an antianxiety medication called buspirone. In some circumstances, your doctor may prescribe benzodiazepines—such as Xanax (alprazolam), Valium (diazepam), or Ativan (lorazepam)—to relieve symptoms of acute anxiety on a short-term basis, but these can be habit-forming, so they should be used with caution.

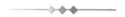

There's no question that minding your moods is incredibly important for your physical and psychological health as well as your overall quality of life. But you may not have realized (until now) the extent to which depression and anxiety, in particular, drain your energy and lead to exhaustion. This is yet another reason why it's important to seek medical attention if you have fatigue without other symptoms: It may be a sign of depression or anxiety, even if you don't have the usual telltale signs of either condition. Exploring possible reasons for your fatigue, along with your underlying state of mind, and getting the appropriate treatment for a mental-health disorder can boost your mood and restore your vim and vigor. There's nothing but an upside here.

PART IV

Repairing Your

Energy Drains

CHAPTER FOURTEEN

Your Personalized Energy-Boosting Plan

BY NOW, YOU'VE ASSESSED your relative exhaustion and energy levels. You've read about the lifestyle factors that can contribute to, worsen, or improve your fatigue, and you've learned about various medical conditions that slowly and insidiously drain your energy. Now it's time to unmask the true source(s) of *your* exhaustion and find ways to break out of your lethargy and reclaim your vitality. In other words, it's time to put together a personalized energy-boosting plan that's likely to work for you. This may seem easier said than done, but if you approach this task in a systematic fashion, you will begin to solve your personal energy crisis one step at a time.

As a starting point, I recommend doing a 7-day fatigue-beating challenge— a preliminary intervention that addresses the most common factors that play a role in chronic exhaustion. It's going to take some time to implement these measures, so it's best to undertake this challenge during a week when you can lighten your usual schedule and responsibilities. The approach employs eight strategies that are likely to benefit all women and help tease out the roots of their exhaustion, thereby setting the stage for additional interventions to address their unique issues. The goal is to incorporate these strategies into your daily regimen for a week and then to reassess your fatigue. My hope is that you'll notice at least some improvement after just 7 days. Let's get started!

1. Keep a Fatigue Diary

Before you can learn to manage your exhaustion, you need to find out what triggers it, what makes it worse, and what factors seem to reduce it. One of the best ways to pinpoint your fatigue patterns is to keep a daily diary, in which you rate the quality and quantity of your sleep from the night before, jot down what you eat and drink (and when you do it), note your physical activities throughout the day, monitor your stress level throughout the day, and track the ebb and flow of your energy.

You'll find a sample fatigue diary in Appendix A. The chart has vertical columns for the days of the week and horizontal rows with spaces in which you can track your diet and exercise patterns, your stress and energy levels, and more. Once you've completed a chart for a week, you'll get an unvarnished look at what's really going on with your lifestyle habits and your fatigue cycles throughout each day. Take a close look at the patterns: Are there consistent peaks and valleys in your energy level during your waking hours? Can you detect any factors that consistently make your exhaustion better or worse?

Some women find that monitoring their lifestyle habits, stress levels, and energy-versus-fatigue patterns is helpful in itself because it puts them back in touch with their bodies and places their symptoms in a more realistic light. They might come to realize, for example, that they're not really exhausted 24/7 as they thought they were but that their energy and fatigue levels have highs and lows throughout the day. They might discover powerful connections between their sedentary habits or their stress levels and their exhaustion. Or they might realize that making small alterations to their lifestyle habits—tweaking what they eat for breakfast or lunch, or taking a brisk walk—can make a considerable difference in their subsequent energy level.

2. Sleep Solo

Even if you're married or in a committed relationship, try sleeping alone during the 7-day fatigue challenge to prevent other people from affecting the quality of your shut-eye. Of course, you can have conjugal activities, but then retreat to your own bed and room. The goal is to literally and figuratively close the door and not be bothered by anyone else's sleep patterns. Your partner will forgive you; in fact, he or she will probably love you even more if you're less tired!

Dedicate at least 8 hours to sleep each night, in a room that's cool, dark, and quiet. At least half an hour before bed, turn off your computer and the TV, and charge your mobile phone in another room. Scan the bedroom for blinking or glowing lights (from the alarm clock, the DVD clock and timer, and so on)—turn these off or cover the displays. Every little bit of light exposure can prevent your melatonin levels from rising as they should in the evening; you need melatonin to fall sleep and to reach the deep restorative stages of sleep that your body requires. If you can't darken your room all the way, wear a sleep mask or install blackout curtains or shades.

Before turning in for the night, consider taking a magnesium supplement to help you relax before bed and get a sounder night's sleep. (I like a product called Natural Calm, which contains calcium and magnesium in powder form; you simply add water and drink it.) You also may want to add a supplement of 5-HTP, an amino acid the body uses to produce serotonin, a calming neurotransmitter that helps improve sleep quality. Also, if you're already on them, continue taking sleep aids at the same time every night—good-quality sleep relies on consistent habits! Before turning in for the night, spend a few minutes doing deep breathing, muscle relaxation exercises, or calming yoga poses. You might try soaking in a magnesium-rich Epsom salt bath before bed to help reduce muscle tension, relax your blood vessels, and set you up for a good night's sleep. Simply pour 1 cup of Epsom salts and 1 cup of baking soda into a warm bath, then have a good soak an hour before slipping between the sheets.

3. Stick with a Clean Diet

That means no processed foods for 7 days. Consume only whole foods that are in their recognizable form (as in vegetables, fruits, 100 percent whole grains, nuts, seeds, beans, legumes, and lean protein). Avoid simple sugars—not just table sugar but also syrups and anything that has an ingredient that ends in *-ose,* such as glucose, sucrose, maltose, and dextrose. To keep things easy, try following this rule of thumb: If an item has an ingredients label, don't eat it. Also, drink minimal, if any, alcohol, and keep your caffeine intake on the low side (don't quit cold turkey, though—doing so may trigger rebound headaches and more fatigue).

Have one "green drink" per day, ideally for breakfast or before noon. To supercharge your energy reserves, you can't beat green drinks: They deliver concentrated, high-octane, liquid doses of digestive enzymes and infuse you with phytonutrients and antioxidants—and they do it quickly, easily, and efficiently. These nutrient-rich drinks boost immunity, aid digestion, help keep blood sugar levels steady, sustain energy, promote mental clarity, and enhance overall well-being. You can't ask for much more!

This is my favorite "green drink" recipe (it makes two large glasses, about 20 ounces total):

> *4 green apples, sliced or chopped*
>
> *7–8 large kale leaves (bitter stalks removed)*
>
> *4–5 spinach leaves*
>
> *½ lemon, peeled, seeded, and sliced*
>
> *Water to taste*

Place the ingredients in a juicer or blender and process them until the mixture reaches the desired consistency. Propose a toast to your health, then drink up!

When I'm on the go, I often grab a green drink from Juice Press, a line of retail stores in New York City. In particular, I like "OMG!," which contains celery, cucumber, pear, grapefruit, kale, and parsley juice, and "doctor green juice," which consists of red apple juice, pineapple juice, kale juice, lemon juice, and ginger juice. I realize that people who live outside New

York won't have access to this line of juices, but I'm letting you know my favorite formulas so you can look for something similar in your area or try making your own version at home.

While you're following the clean-eating plan, focus on getting plenty of three nutrients in particular: magnesium, iron, and omega-3 fatty acids. Here's why:

Magnesium: Fatigue is a common sign of a slight magnesium deficiency, which isn't surprising considering that magnesium is needed for more than 300 biochemical reactions in the body, including the breakdown of glucose (from food) into energy. When magnesium levels are even slightly low, your energy level can fall. In a study at the USDA's Grand Forks Human Nutrition Research Center in North Dakota, researchers found that women with even slight magnesium deficiencies had higher heart rates and required more oxygen to perform physical tasks than they did after their magnesium levels were restored to normal. In other words, when your magnesium levels are low, your body ends up working harder than it should have to, which over time may leave you feeling depleted. Besides improving your energy, magnesium plays a role in strengthening your bones and keeps your heart, nerves, muscles, and immune system functioning well. What's more, the mineral can aid in relaxing the muscles surrounding your airways, which helps keep your airways open; this is significant because getting enough oxygen into your lungs and to all your vital organs is essential to feeling energized.

For women, the recommended daily intake of magnesium is around 300 milligrams (it's 350 milligrams for men). You can easily get this by adding a handful of almonds, hazelnuts, sesame seeds, or cashews to your cereal or salad each day; by sprinkling 1 to 2 tablespoons of flaxseeds onto your yogurt (or anything else, really); and by eating fish (especially halibut).

Iron: Some people find that boosting their energy can be as simple as getting more iron in their diets. Iron deficiency is one of the most common nutritional deficiencies and the leading cause of anemia in the United States.

The most common symptom of iron deficiency: fatigue. This mineral is an essential part of hemoglobin, the main component of red blood cells that transfers oxygen from the lungs to the tissues throughout the body. In addition, iron supports metabolism, normal cellular functioning, and the synthesis of some hormones; it's also essential for growth and development.

Women with heavy periods and/or who have a low intake of animal protein and iron-rich veggies (like lentils, spinach, and kale) are most vulnerable to low iron levels (even iron-deficiency anemia). Iron from animal products is absorbed more readily than iron from plant foods, so consider having small servings of organic red meat, poultry, or fish in at least one meal each day during the challenge. If you don't consume animal products and you suspect you can't get enough iron from plant sources or you think your iron level may be low for other reasons, discuss the possibility of taking an iron supplement with your doctor. A 2012 study published in *CMAJ* (*Canadian Medical Association Journal*) found that when premenopausal women with unexplained fatigue (who were low in iron but not anemic) took iron supplements for 12 weeks, their levels of fatigue improved by nearly 50 percent. It's recommended that women between the ages of 19 and 50 consume 18 milligrams of iron per day. After age 51, the average age of menopause (when a woman's periods stop), a woman's iron requirements drop down to 8 milligrams per day.

Omega-3 fatty acids: Many studies have shown that consuming omega-3 fatty acids improves mood and brain function. What's more, these healthy fats—which are found in fish (like salmon, halibut, tuna, lake trout, sardines, and anchovies) as well as flaxseeds, walnuts, canola oil, avocado, and fortified foods—reduce harmful inflammation throughout the body and protect the function and integrity of cell membranes. These effects can add up to a decrease in fatigue and an increase in energy. Try to eat at least one source of omega-3 fatty acids per day during the fatigue challenge.

To keep your blood sugar on an even keel, shift away from having three big meals a day and move toward having five to six balanced mini-meals. That means eating something every 3 to 4 hours during the day. To maintain steady energy levels, it helps to pair complex carbs that are high in fiber (such as beans, peas, and whole grains) with unsaturated fats (such as avocado, walnuts, or mixed greens with olive oil); add some protein (such as lean meat, nuts, fish or seafood, eggs, or edamame) in small portions and you have a balanced mini-meal. Some of my patients find that increasing how often they eat has a substantial energy-boosting effect.

Another dietary measure that's beneficial in the energy department is consuming probiotics, which are present in certain foods (such as yogurt and kefir), capsules and pills, liquids, and chewables. Most products contain lactobacillus or bifidobacterium or acidophilus, all beneficial forms of bacteria that promote good digestive health and a robust metabolism and immune function and that can provide an energy boost in the process. Always check the expiration date to make sure the bacteria in these products are alive and thriving. Some probiotics have "colony forming units" (CFUs) in the billions. The lemon-flavored chewable tablet (BioGaia ProTectis) that I take has around 100 million. (I believe this is adequate for regular maintenance, but you may require more if you're taking antibiotics.) After you buy a probiotic supplement, be sure to protect the package from heat, moisture, and air.

4. Walk for 10 Minutes a Day

Two hours—that's how long you'll feel revved up after taking just a 10-minute walk, according to a 1987 study in the *Journal of Personality and Social Psychology*. In this often-quoted study, Robert Thayer, PhD, professor of psychology at California State University, Long Beach, compared the energizing effects of eating a candy bar to walking briskly for 10 minutes on 12 different days. Walking was the better bet because it increased energy for 2 hours. The sugary snack gave participants an initial boost, but after an hour, they were more tired and had even less energy than they started with. Another study from the same researchers found that when the participants continued the daily 10-minute walks for 3 weeks, their overall energy levels and mood experienced a substantial rise.

My recommendation is to try the 10-minute rule: Make a deal with yourself to get moving for at least 10 minutes. Commit to that, and then see what happens. Chances are, once you start, you'll feel so much better that you'll want to keep going.

5. Check In with Your Body Hourly

Set an alarm to go off every hour and give yourself a brief time-out to survey discomfort in your body. Drop what you're doing, stand up, close your eyes, and focus your mind on the current state of your physical well-being. Starting at the top of your head and working your way down to your feet, examine the sensations in your body, looking for areas of tension, discomfort, or pain. Why do this? Because musculoskeletal pain and tension drain your energy, and many times these sensations are caused or exacerbated by your behavior (slouching in front of a computer, clenching your jaw when you're stressed). This means you can take steps to reverse those contributing factors.

When I was in the throes of my own exhaustion crisis, this exercise became a welcome ritual for me: I often talked to myself out loud as I did it. For example, I'd say, "Is my scalp tense or itchy?" Moving on to my forehead, I'd ask, "Is my brow furrowed or tense?" Then: "Are my ears ringing, or do they feel full? Am I clenching my jaw? Is my neck uncomfortable or protruding forward instead of being aligned with my shoulder blades? Are my shoulders tensed and hunched up toward my ears, or relaxed and down? What about my chest and breathing?" I would do this all the way down to my feet. Sometimes I would discover that one of my legs had fallen asleep at my desk without my noticing. Once you've done your body-tension inventory, consciously relax any tight areas and focus on shifting positions or activities that are contributing to the discomfort.

This is also a great opportunity to give yourself breathing lessons. We all realize that without breath, there is no life—yet few of us bother to make breathing a conscious activity or think about whether we are breathing well enough to provide our lungs, blood, and brain with enough oxygen to function optimally. Doing the following exercise hourly improves your breathing techniques, so that even when you breathe unconsciously, each breath will be more energizing:

Start by exhaling fully through your mouth, making a whooshing sound with your breath. Then close your mouth and inhale slowly through your nose for 5 seconds. Hold your breath for a count of six, then slowly exhale through your mouth to a count of seven, making that whooshing sound again. Repeat this five times.

Doing breathing exercises like this improves fatigue by calming your nervous system. In fact, a 2011 study from Iran found that when people with chronic obstructive pulmonary disease (COPD) engaged in a regimen of breathing exercises four times a day over a 10-day period, they experienced an average of a 27 percent reduction in the intensity of their fatigue. While this particular study focused on fatigue reversal in COPD patients, the findings also are useful for anyone who is exhausted. Similarly, research from the United Kingdom found that when people engaged in breathing retraining—simply put, they learned to breathe in a more synchronous pattern—they experienced improvements in measures of anxiety and depression.

The next step is to spend 2 to 3 minutes doing some gentle stretches, as follows:

+ **Neck stretch:** With your shoulders down, slowly move your right ear toward your right shoulder—hold this position for 10 seconds, then do the same thing on the left side.

+ **Shoulder stretch:** Place your hands on top of your shoulders, and move your elbows in large circles as you do three big shoulder rolls from the front to the back. Then do three shoulder rolls from the back to the front.

+ **Upper-back stretch:** Clasp your hands in front of you at chest level, maintain a bend in your elbows, round your upper back, and touch your chin to your chest, as if you're giving yourself a big bear hug; hold for 10 seconds.

- **Chest stretch:** Stand in a doorway, facing forward with your feet several inches apart, and grab the sides of the doorframe with your fingers; then push your chest forward until you feel a stretch in your torso and back—hold this position for 15 to 20 seconds.

- **Quad and hip flexor stretch:** Stand with your right foot about 2 feet in front of your left foot, bend your right knee, and lean forward, keeping your torso upright, until you feel a stretch in the front of the left leg and hip; hold for 15 seconds. Switch sides.

- **Hamstring stretch:** Stand with your feet hip-width apart, then move your right foot about 12 to 15 inches forward. Place your left hand on a chair or wall for balance, then place your right heel on the ground and lift your toes. Bend your left knee and reach for your right toes with your right hand. Hold for 10 seconds. Switch sides.

This may sound like a lot to do, but it can all be accomplished in 5 to 7 minutes, and it's worth the effort. After all, the potential payoff is substantial—a reduction in muscle tension and discomfort, an ability to breathe easier and more fully, and a boost in energy. It's time well spent!

6. Drink Water All Day Long

As mentioned earlier, dehydration is one of the most common causes of fatigue, not to mention crankiness and foggy thinking. Even before your thirst mechanism kicks in (typically after your body's hydration level has dropped by 2.6 percent), you'll experience lethargy. This may be because when you're even mildly dehydrated, the fluid loss from your body causes a drop in blood volume, which makes your heart have to work harder to push oxygen and nutrients through the bloodstream to your muscles and organs.

How much water should you drink each day? It's a simple question without an easy answer. Studies have produced varying recommendations over the years, but the truth is, your personal need for water depends on many factors, including your overall health, how active you are, and the climate in which you live. For those who are fighting fatigue, increasing your water intake during the 7-day fatigue-fighting challenge may make a meaningful difference.

The Institute of Medicine determined that an adequate intake for women is about 9 cups (2.2 liters) of total beverages a day and for men it is roughly about 13 cups (3 liters) per day. For energy-boosting purposes, I suggest women take in a minimum of 3 liters daily during this challenge. The easiest way to do this is to buy three 1-liter bottles of water and finish them all by the end of the day. Ideally, you should space out your intake pretty evenly, but of course after exercise you should drink more. Most of all, try not to go an hour without drinking something. If you're not a fan of plain old H_2O, feel free to sip green tea or to add lemon or orange slices to your water—but avoid sugared beverages. Carbonated water is generally fine, but if you're battling any gastrointestinal issues, the bubbly beverages may increase bloating and gas.

While it's an uncommon occurrence, it is possible to drink too much water. When your kidneys are unable to excrete the excess fluids, the electrolyte (mineral) content of your blood becomes diluted, resulting in low sodium levels, which causes the cells to swell—a potentially dangerous condition called hyponatremia. If your kidneys are healthy and functioning properly, don't worry: In general, it's risk-free for most people to consume 3 liters per day.

7. Make a "To-Don't" List

Of course, it's impossible to avoid stress completely, but you may be surprised to discover the number of stressors in your life that you can reduce or eliminate. Making a to-do list is a valuable tool to improve organization, focus, and productivity. But if you're like many women, you may create master or rolling to-do lists that are loaded with tasks that (a) aren't really priorities or (b) don't need to be done by you personally. In that case, the overwhelming list can leave you feeling deflated and defeated because your expectations (or goals) are unrealistic and you're too wiped out to whittle down your list.

The solution: Make a companion "to-don't" list. Of course, hold on to your to-do list and continue adding to it as you see fit—but for the next 7 days, make a point of reevaluating it at least once a day. For each item on the list, ask yourself these three questions:

◆ Am I sure that *I* have to do it and that I can't delegate the task to someone else?

◆ Can the task wait until after the 7-day challenge has been completed (without adding to my stress)?

◆ Can the task be altered to make it simpler and/or less time-consuming?

If the answers to the first two questions are no and yes, respectively, move that item to your to-don't list. If you get to the third question and you can simplify the task, by all means go for it. Meanwhile, for every new item you add to your to-do list, be prepared to move at least one other item (or even two or three) to the to-don't list. The idea is that by setting limits and keeping expectations realistic, you'll be protecting your energy and setting yourself up to accomplish what's crucial. This will lower your stress level and leave you feeling empowered, in turn reducing fatigue. It's an energizing trifecta.

8. Make Sense of Your Symptoms

Once you've completed the 7-day challenge, it's time to reassess your exhaustion. On day 8, compare your fatigue diary from day 7 to the first 2 days of the challenge: How much did your fatigue and its related symptoms improve? Which ones went away completely, which decreased in severity, and which symptoms remain? Do you think some of the steps in the challenge had more of an impact than others did? If so, go back and review the lifestyle chapters on how to improve your sleep, diet, exercise, and/or stress management habits even more so you can get further insight into how to capitalize on the gains you've already begun to make. Then set priorities for what to work on next within the domain that seemed to make the biggest difference for you.

Now it's time to take stock of your long-term symptoms. Use the following checklist to assess them. Circle all the conditions you have experienced within the past year.

GENERAL SYMPTOMS

- Frequently tired
- Always tired
- Loss of appetite
- Unintentional or unexplained weight gain or loss
- Unexplained fever

HEAD SYMPTOMS

- Watery eyes
- Dry eyes
- Itchy eyes
- Seeing spots or flashes of light
- Double vision
- Ear pain
- Ringing in the ears
- Ear drainage
- Hearing loss
- Nasal congestion
- Sinus pressure or pain
- Recurrent sinus infections
- Recurrent colds
- Frequent sore throats
- Hoarseness

HEART AND CIRCULATION SYMPTOMS

- Chest pain or pressure
- Palpitations
- Unexplained rapid heartbeat or irregular heart rate
- High blood pressure

- Leg pain
- Calf cramps
- Swelling of the ankles or feet
- Cold, bluish-red feet

RESPIRATORY SYMPTOMS

- Shortness of breath
- Wheezing
- Persistent cough

- Snoring
- Awakening from sleep gasping for breath

GASTROINTESTINAL SYMPTOMS

- Frequent nausea
- Unexplained vomiting
- Heartburn
- Bloating after meals
- Cramping during digestion

- Bloody stool
- Recurrent diarrhea
- Recurrent constipation
- Hemorrhoids

GENITOURINARY SYMPTOMS

- Pain on urination
- Difficulty starting urination
- Waking up to urinate during the night
- Irregular periods

- Heavy periods
- Vaginal discharge or itching
- Loss of sex drive

MUSCULOSKELETAL SYMPTOMS

- Joint pain/stiffness
- General muscle aches
- Pain in the neck or back
- Elbow or shoulder pain
- Hand or wrist pain
- Pain in the ankles or feet

SKIN SYMPTOMS

- Unexplained rash
- Dry skin
- Itching
- Hives
- Change in skin color

NEUROLOGIC SYMPTOMS

- Headaches
- Fainting
- Dizziness or light-headedness
- Changes in balance or coordination
- Tremors
- Memory loss
- Problems remembering words
- Numbness in the limbs

MENTAL-HEALTH SYMPTOMS

- Anxiety
- Depressed feelings
- Poor attention span
- Excess fear or worry
- Loss of interest in normally enjoyable activities
- Suicidal thoughts
- Difficulty concentrating
- Difficulty getting to sleep or staying asleep
- Impulsivity

ENDOCRINE SYMPTOMS

- Always feel cold
- Always feel hot
- Facial hair growth
- Hair loss

- Excessive thirst
- Excessive urination
- Excessive sweating
- Hot flashes

Look over the symptoms you've circled. Items under General Symptoms should be noted and brought to the attention of your doctor. If you have more than three in any category, refer to the corresponding chapter related to those symptoms. If you marked three or more symptoms under:

- "Head," review Chapter 11.
- "Heart and Circulation" or "Respiratory," consult Chapter 9.
- "Gastrointestinal," see Chapter 10.
- "Genitourinary," consult Chapters 7 and 11.
- "Musculoskeletal," turn to Chapters 8 and 12.
- "Skin" or "Endocrine," see Chapters 7 and 8.
- "Neurologic," consult Chapters 11, 12, and 13.
- "Mental Health," see Chapter 13.

Your next step is to make an appointment with your physician for a thorough physical examination and perhaps a battery of lab tests. Bring a copy of your symptom checklist and your fatigue diary with you to the appointment. This offers your doctor a clear view of your recent symptoms, a glimpse into your energy-fatigue cycles, and a sense of how your lifestyle habits may contribute to your fatigue. My hope is that armed with this information, you and your doctor can take a big step forward on your journey toward ending exhaustion and reigniting your energy.

Five Quick Tricks to Boost Your Energy

While you're trying to get to the bottom of your energy crisis and taking long-term steps to reverse it, don't hesitate to jump-start your energy for even a short time. Every little boost counts, and the more productive you can be, the more empowered you're likely to feel. Here are five tried-and-true ways to pump up your energy when you need a boost most.

CHECK YOUR POSTURE. While gazing at the floor from a standing position, you should be able to see the tops of your shoes without craning your neck. Another quick alignment check: In a standing or sitting position, your head should be lined up over, not in front of, your body so that your ears are directly over your shoulders. Why do this? Slouching doesn't just make you look tired—it makes you feel tired, too, because it places excess strain on your back and hips; plus, when your joints aren't properly aligned, your whole body has to work harder than it should. Additionally, standing or sitting tall will improve the flow of oxygen to your brain, which increases your alertness and attentiveness.

EXPOSE YOURSELF TO LIGHT. Throw open the curtains and sit in a sunny window or step outside periodically. Environmental cues play a huge role in the body's energy cycles throughout the day, and regular exposure to natural light has been shown to maintain higher energy levels in people suffering from fatigue. Exposure to natural sunlight can also enhance your mood. If you work in a windowless environment, try to step outside for some light therapy for 5 minutes every hour if possible.

USE GOOD SCENTS. This isn't about dousing yourself with your favorite perfume. It's about harnessing the power of aromatherapy to lift your spirits when you need it. Take a whiff of peppermint, rosemary, or jasmine when you feel droopy—research shows these scents increase alertness. (By contrast, lavender oil and the pure scent of vanilla have relaxing effects on both your physical and emotional states.)

SURROUND YOURSELF WITH ENERGIZING COLORS. Focusing your eyes on a vibrant shade of red, orange, or yellow has an energy-boosting effect on the body, partly because these hues represent heat and radiant energy (think fire, sun). So tie a red, orange, or yellow scarf loosely around your neck so you can see it or place a vase of blooms in these colors on your desk.

GIVE YOURSELF THE RIGHT SOUND TRACK. Numerous studies have found that listening to pleasant music lowers blood pressure, reduces stress, and improves mood. Plus, unplugging from melatonin-suppressing TV and computer screens will improve your ability to fall asleep when your head hits the pillow. So use music strategically: While listening to slower tunes can alter brain activity in a way that leads to a reduction in stress and pain, tuning in to upbeat music that has a high beat-per-minute count (120 or higher) can rev up your energy when you need it (during a workout, for example).

Conclusion

HOPEFULLY, AFTER READING THIS book, you'll have begun to reclaim some of your lost energy through lifestyle changes. Or at least you'll have found a possible link between your fatigue and a medical condition that can be treated with your doctor's help. By now, you probably realize that even if you are fortunate to have a doctor whom you trust and have faith in, you're in the driver's seat on your personal journey to feeling more vibrant, energized, and fulfilled. If your primary-care physician doesn't help you get to the bottom of your exhaustion, see another doctor or ask for a referral to a specialist, based on your constellation of symptoms and fatigue patterns. It's your body and your energy—you're the only one who can persist until you find a remedy for what's making you so tired. And I urge you to do just that!

Fatigue is often viewed as an inevitable side effect of a busy woman's life, especially if she works outside the home and has children, but it doesn't have to be. Don't wave the white flag and accept your exhaustion as a fact of modern life. *Fight it!* But don't judge it, either; it's not a sign that you're not capable enough or disciplined enough. It's a sign that you're tired and that your body is out of balance in some way—and that it's time to take action to remedy that reality. There's no good reason why you should continue running on empty or feeling bedraggled, depleted, or downright wiped out.

It truly is within your power to revive, recharge, and revitalize yourself. You can reclaim your energy and vitality, but it will take some time, attention, and effort on your part.

I assure you: It will be worth the investment. This is your life and your well-being that we're talking about. If you take steps now to cultivate, protect, and nurture your energy, it will return the favor by a factor of 10 in the future. With greater vim and vigor, you'll feel and function better, you'll be less stressed, healthier, and more able to lead the life you want. You deserve to feel robust and vibrant, to enjoy life fully, and to become the best version of yourself that you can be. Give yourself that gift.

I hope that at the very least this book has served as a wake-up call (so to speak) and as a source of inspiration that it's time to unchain yourself from the shackles of fatigue, kick your exhaustion to the curb, and get on with the business of living well and feeling good. Let the dietary, exercise, and stress- and sleep-management strategies in these pages serve as stepping-stones to bring you closer to greater vitality, well-being, empowerment, and fulfillment. As time goes on, you'll want to tweak the advice in this book to make it work for you and your personal needs. Don't be afraid to personalize my suggestions; it's been my intention all along that you would. Every woman is different—we have different bodies, different health profiles, varying circumstances, personalities, aspirations, and so on—so we each need to find strategies that effectively address our individual needs. There's no one-size-fits-all solution here.

Keep in mind: Your exhaustion breakthrough and your ongoing energy management plan will be a continuous work in progress. Don't be surprised if even after you've started to gain a grip on your fatigue and reverse it, you experience occasional setbacks with flare-ups of exhaustion. When that happens, consider it your body's signal that you may be overextending yourself or relapsing into habits that sabotage your energy. View it as a warning sign that you need to honor and respect your limits, and perhaps hit the pause button or cut back on certain obligations so that you can devote more time to taking better care of yourself.

I see this waxing-and-waning phenomenon play out all the time with patients in my practice—and in my personal life. The truth is, my own fatigue-fighting odyssey continues to be a work in progress. I have good periods and not-so-good periods, better months and worse months—but I can honestly say that I've come a long way from my low ebb. These days, I'm usually at a 7 or an 8 on a scale of 1 to 10, with 10 being high energy—that's pretty good, all things considered.

There isn't anything in this book that I haven't tried; some interventions worked for me, others didn't. Thanks to a process of trial and error, I have found a fatigue-fighting formula—a combination of traditional and alternative treatments and lifestyle modifications—that benefits me, and I stick with it. If I skip my power walks and my green juice for a few days, I really feel it. I have also learned to heed my limits; I try not to overcommit myself even within a high level of professional and personal activities and obligations. I have learned how to say no to requests and invitations that are too much for me: If there's a 9 o'clock dinner, for example, no matter how special it is, I can't do it. There are people who can, but I'm not one of them. I have developed a keen sense of what's doable and what's not for me—and I try to live within those boundaries. I think this has made a difference in my overall energy level and my sense of well-being.

My life circumstances haven't changed dramatically. My days are still packed with various activities from morning to night. I seldom get an uninterrupted night's sleep. And I often end up taking work-related phone calls on the fly or on the fire escape of my New York apartment, where I can be out of range of my lovable but spirited children. The important thing is that I have discovered energy-boosting solutions that are effective for me. Because I've done that, I'm not just able to handle the pressure and chaos of my hectic life—I embrace them. These days, I enjoy life more than ever—and I feel like I'm thriving once again. My hope is that once you discover what's draining your energy and which treatments restore your vim and vigor, your energy crisis will come to an end and you'll begin to thrive again, too. You deserve nothing less than that.

Appendix A: Fatigue Diary

DAY OF THE WEEK			MONDAY	TUESDAY	WEDNESDAY	
Sleep quality—previous night*						
Sleep duration						
Energy assessment*		7 a.m.				
		10 a.m.				
		1 p.m.				
		4 p.m.				
		7 p.m.				
		10 p.m.				
Meals—time and quality+		Breakfast				
		Lunch				
		Dinner				
		Snacks				
Water intake—time/amount						
Physical activity*		9 a.m.				
		12 noon				
		3 p.m.				
		6 p.m.				
		9 p.m.				
Stress level*		7 a.m.				
		10 a.m.				
		1 p.m.				
		4 p.m.				
		7 p.m.				
		10 p.m.				
Notes to self:						
Things I suspect made fatigue better						
Things I suspect made fatigue worse						

*Rate the quality on a scale from 1 to 10, with 1 being low (as in poor sleep, low energy, low physical activity, high stress) and 10 being high (excellent sleep, high energy, lots of physical activity, low stress).
+Rate your food choices as poor, fair, good, or excellent in terms of nutritional quality.

	THURSDAY	FRIDAY	SATURDAY	SUNDAY

Medications That Can Make You Tired

WHEN YOU TAKE A medication for a chronic health problem, you expect it to make you feel better—and it often does. Sometimes, though, a medication-driven improvement in one health condition comes at a cost, namely in the form of side effects. One common side effect that's often overlooked is fatigue. That's right: Ongoing fatigue (including lethargy and/ or listlessness) is often an adverse effect of drugs that are prescribed for other conditions. Here's a look at eight of the most common culprits.

1. **Antibiotics:** Many different classes of antibiotics are used to treat infections or conditions caused by bacteria, and it's long been recognized that some people experience noticeable fatigue or lethargy while they're on the drugs. The reasons for this aren't clear, but it's a widely recognized phenomenon; that's why you'll often see fatigue, tiredness, or weakness listed as potential side effects on the package inserts of these prescription medications.

2. **Antidepressants:** There are many different types of antidepressants, including selective serotonin reuptake inhibitors (SSRIs), serotonin and norepinephrine reuptake inhibitors (SNRIs), tricyclic antidepressants, and others. Fatigue is a common side effect with many of them, especially as your body is adjusting to the medication in the first few weeks. This may result from the drugs' effects on neurotransmitters (brain chemicals), such as serotonin and norepinephrine, and hormones (including stress hormones).

3. **Antihistamines:** These drugs—often used to treat allergies, colds, motion sickness, and insomnia—depress the central nervous system, which is why drowsiness, fatigue, and weakness are possible side effects (they're often listed on the package). Some of the newer generation antihistamines, such as loratadine and cetirizine, are less likely to cause fatigue.

4. **Antipsychotics:** Used to treat schizophrenia, bipolar disorder, and other serious psychiatric conditions, antipsychotic drugs have a powerful depressant effect on the central nervous system. As a result, side effects such as fatigue, lethargy, and weakness are common. Some of these drugs also lower levels of the neurotransmitter dopamine, which can lead to drowsiness and sleepiness.

5. **Benzodiazepines:** There's a reason why they're also known as tranquilizers—benzodiazepines (like Xanax, Klonopin, and Ativan) have sedating effects and cause fatigue by reducing activity in key parts of the central nervous system. They're used to treat anxiety, agitation, and sometimes insomnia, as well as to prevent seizures.

6. **Blood-pressure medications:** ACE inhibitors, beta-blockers, and calcium channel blockers may result in fatigue by slowing down the heart's pumping action and depressing the central nervous system. By contrast, diuretics deplete vitamins, minerals, and fluids that your body relies on for energy, and they can interfere with the balance of electrolytes (including sodium, potassium, and chloride) in your body, causing weakness.

7. **Cholesterol-lowering medications:** Statins and fibrates, both used to treat high cholesterol, are linked with fatigue because they interfere with the production of energy at the cellular level and reduce production of satellite cells in the muscles, thereby retarding muscle growth. (Muscle weakness is a frequent side effect of statins.)

8. **Proton pump inhibitors:** Used to treat gastroesophageal reflux disease, chronic heartburn, and peptic ulcers, proton pump inhibitors (PPIs) reduce the amount of acid your stomach makes. Taking PPIs for 3 months or longer may result in low blood levels of magnesium, which causes fatigue and lethargy among other symptoms.

If you think your tiredness might be linked to a medication you're taking, don't stop taking it. Talk to your doctor about the possible connection and what you might be able to do about it. In some cases, tinkering with the time of day that you take the drug or changing the dose can make a significant difference; in other instances, switching to another drug might be the answer.

APPENDIX C

Energy-Boosting Supplements

WE'RE A COUNTRY THAT loves quick fixes, which partly explains why energy-enhancing supplements have become one of the fastest-growing categories of nutritional products on the market. Yet the reality is, with many of these so-called energy boosters, there's little scientific evidence to prove their effectiveness (as in the case of bee pollen, royal jelly, and others). Others (like bitter orange, a compound similar to ephedra or ma huang, which has been banned in the United States) can have dangerous side effects like heart palpitations and elevated blood pressure. But some popular supplements do have a respectable amount of science behind them to support their use for a brief boost in energy—and those are the ones I want to focus on. Here's a look at what they are and how they work.

STIMULATING PLANTS

Yes, it's true: **Caffeine** really can rev you up. It does, in fact, increase resting metabolic rate, causing you to burn calories at a slightly faster rate than usual, and it increases alertness and concentration for a while. It does all this by stimulating the central nervous system (which in turn causes the heart to supply more oxygen-rich blood to the cells), by increasing energy metabolism in the brain, and by triggering the release of the neurotransmitter dopamine. In addition to coffee and tea, herbal sources of caffeine include guarana, yerba mate, and kola nut. The downside is, caffeine can be habit forming, and if you consume it in excess, you may require higher doses to achieve the same effect.

Green tea is another stimulant, in part because it contains caffeine as well as a related compound called theophylline and also because it contains a powerful antioxidant called epigallocatechin gallate (EGCG). It's EGCG, in particular, that may have unique effects on mental and physical energy, effects that are greater than those from caffeine alone. New research suggests, for example, that EGCG enhances mitochondrial function and protects against mitochondrial damage, which is significant because the mitochondria are the batteries or power sources in our cells.

In addition, some herbs and spices have stimulating effects. **Capsaicin,** a compound that gives chile peppers their heat, is thought to enhance blood circulation and provide a brief, but mild, metabolic boost. It can also relieve pain when it's applied topically (in a cream, for example). But it isn't used much for direct improvements in physical or mental energy.

By contrast, **Asian ginseng** stimulates the central nervous system and increases resistance to fatigue. Known as an adaptogen, this herb helps the body adapt to increased levels of stress. It has been used to increase well-being and stamina and to improve mental and physical performance, though it has not been widely studied for these uses. The herb has adverse interactions with some prescription drugs, so it's important to consult your doctor before adding this to your regimen.

NUTRITIONAL BOOSTS

A handful of vitamins and other nutrients may relieve fatigue by affecting your metabolism—namely, how your cells derive energy from nutrients. **Coenzyme Q10**, for example, is a natural substance that's found in mitochondria, and it's involved in the synthesis of adenosine triphosphate (ATP), the major energy source of cells. In theory, coenzyme Q10 increases energy by providing cells with more ATP. Certain medications and/or a nutrient-poor diet can lead to a deficiency of coenzyme Q10, in which case supplements may be particularly beneficial.

Eight different B vitamins play a role in the production of energy within the cells, but **B₆, B₁₂, folic acid, niacin,** and **thiamin** are especially important. Low levels or borderline deficiencies in these B vitamins are more common than you might think. Those who are especially susceptible include people who consume diets high in processed foods, those who take regular medications (such as acid blockers for gastroesophageal reflux disease or anti-inflammatory painkillers), and athletes who train hard. Before supplementing selectively, have your blood levels of these nutrients tested.

A variety of amino acids—including creatine, carnitine, taurine, tyrosine, and others—play a role in the synthesis of protein. Two amino acids are especially important in the energy department: **Creatine** helps build muscle and reduce fatigue by transporting extra energy into your cells, whereas **carnitine** is involved in energy production in mitochondria inside the cells. As helpful as they may be, supplements of these nutrients also come with potential side effects—such as water retention and gastrointestinal upset—so talk to your doctor before you try them.

The bottom line with supplements: More isn't necessarily better. Even though most supplements are derived from compounds found in nature, they can have potentially detrimental effects, especially if you have an underlying health condition or take other medications. So, please, consult your physician before you start swallowing supplements to boost your energy.

Selected Reading

Ahola, K., I. Sirén, M. Kivimaki, S. Ripatti, A. Aromaa, J. Lonnqvist, and I. Hovatta. "Work-Related Exhaustion and Telomere Length: A Population-Based Study." *PLoS One* 7, no. 7 (2012): e40186.

Ament, W., and G. J. Verkerke. "Exercise and Fatigue." *Sports Medicine* 39, no. 5 (2009): 389–422.

American Psychological Association. "Stress in America: Missing the Health Care Connection." 2012.

Ando, M., T. Morita, T. Akechi, S. Ito, M. Tanaka, Y. Ifuku, and T. Nakayama. "The Efficacy of Mindfulness-Based Meditation Therapy on Anxiety, Depression, and Spirituality in Japanese Patients with Cancer." *Journal of Palliative Medicine* 12, no. 12 (December 2009): 1091–94.

Behan, P. O., W. M. Behan, and D. Horrobin. "Effect of High Doses of Essential Fatty Acids on the Postviral Fatigue Syndrome." *Acta Neurologica Scandinavica* 82, no. 3 (September 1990): 209–16.

Bellingrath, S., T. Weigl, and B. M. Kudiekla. "Chronic Work Stress and Exhaustion Is Associated with Higher Allostastic Load in Female School Teachers." *Stress* 12, no. 1 (January 2009): 37–48.

Bjørk, C. Petersen, A. Bauman, M. Grønbaek, J. Wulff Helge, L. C. Thygesen, and J. S. Tolstrup. "Total Sitting Time and Risk of Myocardial Infarction, Coronary Heart Disease and All-Cause Mortality in a Prospective Cohort of Danish Adults." *International Journal of Behavioral Nutrition and Physical Activity* 11, no. 13 (February 5, 2014): 1479–5868.

Bjornsdottir, S., S. Jonsson, and U. Valdimarsdottir. "Mental Health Indicators and Quality of Life among Individuals with Musculoskeletal Chronic Pain: A Nationwide Study in Iceland." *Scandinavian Journal of Rheumatology* 43, no. 5 (2014): 419–23.

Bowen, R., L. Balbuena, M. Baetz, and L. Schwartz. "Maintaining Sleep and Physical Activity Alleviate Mood Instability." *Preventive Medicine* 57, no. 5 (November 2013): 461–65.

Brimmer, D. J., F. Fridinger, S. L. Jin-Mann, and W. C. Reeves. "U.S. Healthcare Providers' Knowledge, Attitudes, Beliefs, and Perceptions Concerning Chronic Fatigue Syndrome." *BMC Family Practice* 11, no. 1 (2010): 28.

Buman, M. P., M. A. Phillips, S. D. Youngstedt, C. E. Kline, and M. Hirshkowitz. "Does Nighttime Exercise Really Disturb Sleep? Results from the 2013 National Sleep Foundation Sleep in America Poll." *Sleep Medicine* 15, no. 7 (July 2014): 755–61.

Buskila, D., J. N. Ablin, I. Ben-Zion, D. Muntanu, A. Shaley, P. Sarzi-Puttini, and H. Cohen. "A Painful Train of Events: Increased Prevalence of Fibromyalgia in Survivors of a Major Train Crash." *Clinical and Experimental Rheumatology* 27, no. 5, Supplement 56 (September–October 2009): S79–85.

Canivet, C., P. O. Ostergren, S. I. Lindeberg, B. Choi, R. Karasek, M. Moghaddassi, and S. O. Isaccson. "Conflict between the Work and Family Domains and Exhaustion among Vocationally Active Men and Women." *Social Science & Medicine* 70, no. 8 (April 2010): 1237–45.

Centers for Disease Control and Prevention. "QuickStats: Percentage of Adults Who Often Felt Very Tired or Exhausted in the Past 3 Months, by Sex and Age Group—National Health Interview Survey, United States, 2010–2011." *Morbidity and Mortality Weekly Report (MMWR)* 62, no. 14 (April 12, 2013): 275.

Christodoulou, C. "The Assessment and Measurement of Fatigue." In *Fatigue as a Window to the Brain.* Edited by John DeLuca. Cambridge: MIT Press, 2005.

Cope, H. "Fatigue: A Non-Specific Complaint?" *International Review of Psychiatry* 4, no. 3 (1992): 273–79.

Dailey, D. L., V. J. Keffala, and K. A. Sluka. "Do Cognitive and Physical Fatigue Tasks Enhance Pain, Cognitive Fatigue, and Physical Fatigue in People with Fibromyalgia?" *Arthritis Care & Research* 67, no. 2 (February 2015): 288–96.

Davis, M. C., M. A. Okun, D. Kruszewski, A. J. Zautra, and H. Tennen. "Sex Differences in the Relations of Positive and Negative Daily Events and Fatigue in Adults with Rheumatoid Arthritis." *The Journal of Pain* 11, no. 12 (December 2010): 1338–47.

DeLuca, J. "Fatigue: Its Definition, Its Study, and Its Future." In *Fatigue as a Window to the Brain.* Edited by John DeLuca. Cambridge: MIT Press, 2005.

Dishman, R. K., N. J. Thom, T. W. Puetz, P. J. O'Connor, and B. A. Clementz. "Effects of Cycling Exercise on Vigor, Fatigue, and Electroencephalographic Activity among Young Adults Who Report Persistent Fatigue." *Psychophysiology* 47, no. 6 (November 2010): 1066–74.

Dittner, A. J., S. C. Wessely, and R. G. Brown. "The Assessment of Fatigue: A Practical Guide for Clinicians and Researchers." *Journal of Psychosomatic Research* 56, no. 2 (2004): 157–70.

Dobrosoielski, D. A., S. Patil, A. R. Schwartz, K. Bandeen-Roche, and K. J. Stewart. "Effects of Exercise and Weight Loss in Older Adults with Obstructive Sleep Apnea." *Medicine and Science in Sports and Exercise* 47, no. 1 (January 2015): 20–26.

Durcan, L., F. Wilson, and G. Cunnane. "The Effect of Exercise on Sleep and Fatigue in Rheumatoid Arthritis: A Randomized Controlled Study." *Journal of Rheumatology* 41, no. 10 (October 2014): 1966–73.

Edlund, M. *The Power of Rest: Why Sleep Alone Is Not Enough.* New York: HarperOne, 2010.

Fava, M., S. Ball, J. C. Nelson, J. Sparks, T. Konechnik, P. Classi, S. Dube, and M. E. Thase. "Clinical Relevance of Fatigue as a Residual Symptom in Major Depressive Disorder." *Depression and Anxiety* 31, no. 3 (March 2014): 250–57.

Fetzner, M. G., and G. J. Asmundson. "Aerobic Exercise Reduces Symptoms of Posttraumatic Stress Disorder: A Randomized Controlled Trial." *Cognitive Behaviour Therapy,* June 9, 2013, 1–13.

Floderus, B., M. Hagman, G. Aronsson, S. Marklund, and A. Wikman. "Work Status, Work Hours and Health in Women with and without Children." *Occupational and Environmental Medicine* 66, no. 10 (October 2009): 704–10.

Foster, J. A. "Gut Feelings: Bacteria and the Brain." *Cerebrum* July–August 2013, 9.

Fritschi, C., L. Quinn, E. D. Hacker, S. M. Penckofer, E. Wang, M. Foreman, and C. E. Ferrans. "Fatigue in Women with Type 2 Diabetes." *The Diabetes Educator* 38, no. 5 (September–October 2012): 662–72.

Fukuda, K. "An Epidemiologic Study of Fatigue with Relevance for the Chronic Fatigue Syndrome." *Journal of Psychiatric Research* 31, no. 1 (1997): 19–29.

Garcia, M. N., A. M. Hause, C. M. Walker, J. S. Orange, R. Hasbun, and K. O. Murray. "Evaluation of Prolonged Fatigue Post-West Nile Virus Infection and Association of Fatigue with Elevated Antiviral and Proinflammatory Cytokines." *Viral Immunology* 27, no. 7 (September 2014): 327–33.

Gerrits, M. M., P. van Oppen, S. S. Leone, H. W. van Marwiik, H. E. van der Horst, and B. W. Penninx. "Pain, Not Chronic Disease, Is Associated with the Recurrence of Depressive and Anxiety Disorders." *BMC Psychiatry* 14, June 25, 2014, 187.

Glise, K., G. Ahlborg Jr., and I. H. Jonsdottir. "Course of Mental Symptoms in Patients with Stress-Related Exhaustion: Does Sex or Age Make a Difference?" *BMC Psychiatry* 12, March 12, 2012, 18.

Glise, K., G. Ahlborg Jr., and I. H. Jonsdottir. "Prevalence and Course of Somatic Symptoms in Patients with Stress-Related Exhaustion: Does Sex or Age Matter." *BMC Psychiatry* 12, April 23, 2014, 118.

Gudleski, G. D., and G. D. Shean. "Depressed and Nondepressed Students: Differences in Interpersonal Perceptions." *Journal of Psychology* 134, no. 1 (January 2000): 56–62.

Hambrook, D., A. Oldershaw, K. Rimes, U. Schmidt, K. Tchanturia, J. Treasure, S. Richards, and T. Chalder. "Emotional Expression, Self-Silencing, and Distress Tolerance in Anorexia Nervosa and Chronic Fatigue Syndrome." *The British Journal of Clinical Psychology* 50, no. 3 (September 2011): 310–25.

Handley, A. K., S. J. Egan, R. T. Kane, and C. S. Rees. "The Relationships between Perfectionism, Pathological Worry and Generalised Anxiety Disorder." *BMC Psychiatry* 14, April 2, 2014, 98.

Hauser, W., A. Galek, B. Erbsloh-Moller, V. Kollner, H. Kuhn-Becker, J. Langhorst, F. Petermann, U. Prothmann, A. Winkelmann, G. Schmutzer, E. Brahler, and H. Glaesmer. "Posttraumatic Stress Disorder in Fibromyalgia Syndrome: Prevalence, Temporal Relationship between Posttraumatic Stress and Fibromyalgia Symptoms, and Impact on Clinical Outcome." *Pain* 154, no. 8 (August 2013): 1216–23.

Herring, M. P., and P. J. O'Connor. "The Effect of Acute Resistance Exercise on Feelings of Energy and Fatigue." *Journal of Sports Sciences* 27, no. 7 (May 2009): 701–9.

Hickie, I., T. Davenport, D. Wakefield, U. Vollmer-Conna, B. Cameron, S. D. Vernon, W. C. Reeves, and A. Lloyd. "Post-Infective and Chronic Fatigue Syndromes Precipitated by Viral and Non-Viral Pathogens: Prospective Cohort Study." *BMJ* 333, no. 7568 (September 16, 2006): 575.

Hoffman, B. M., M. A. Babyak, W. E. Craighead, A. Sherwood, P. M. Doraiswamy, M. J. Coons, and J. A. Blumenthal. "Exercise and Pharmacotherapy in Patients with Major Depression: One-Year Follow-Up of the SMILE Study." *Psychosomatic Medicine* 73, no. 2 (February–March 2011): 127–33.

Jackson, M. L., E. M. Sztendur, N. T. Diamond, J. E. Byles, and D. Bruck. "Sleep Difficulties and the Development of Depression and Anxiety: A Longitudinal Study of Young Australian Women." *Archives of Women's Mental Health* 17, no. 3 (June 2014): 189–98.

Johns, S. A., L. F. Brown, K. Beck-Coon, P. O. Monahan, Y. Tong, and K. Kroenke. "Randomized Controlled Pilot Study of Mindfulness-Based Stress Reduction for Persistently

Fatigued Cancer Survivors." *Psychooncology,* August 17, 2014. doi: 10.1002/pon.3648. [Epub ahead of print]

Jones, D. E., J. C. Gray, and J. Newton. "Perceived Fatigue Is Comparable between Different Disease Groups." *QJM* 102, no. 9 (September 2009): 617–24.

Junghaenel, D. U., C. Christodoulou, J. S. Lai, and A. A. Stone. "Demographic Correlates of Fatigue in the US General Population: Results from the Patient-Reported Outcomes Measurement Information System (PROMIS) Initiative." *Journal of Psychosomatic Research* 71, no. 3 (September 2011): 117–23.

Kaleth, A. S., J. E. Slaven, and D. C. Ang. "Increasing Steps/Day Predicts Improvement in Physical Function and Pain Interference in Adults with Fibromyalgia." *Arthritis Care & Research,* July 21, 2014. doi: 10.1002/acr.22398. [Epub ahead of print]

Kiecolt-Glaser, J. K., J. M. Bennett, R. Andridge, J. Peng, C. L. Shapiro, W. B. Malarkey, C. F. Emery, R. Layman, E. E. Mrozek, and R. Glaser. "Yoga's Impact on Inflammation, Mood, and Fatigue in Breast Cancer Survivors: A Randomized Controlled Trial." *Journal of Clinical Oncology* 32, no. 10 (April 1, 2014): 1040–49.

Kim, H. S., M. J. Quon, and J. Kim. "New Insights into the Mechanisms of Polyphenols beyond Antioxidant Properties; Lessons from the Green Tea Polyphenol, Epigallocatechin 3-Gallate." *Redox Biology* 2, January 10, 2014, 187–95.

Lane, T. J., D. A. Matthews, and P. Manu. "The Low Yield of Physical Examinations and Laboratory Investigations of Patients with Chronic Fatigue." *The American Journal of the Medical Sciences* 299, no. 5 (1990): 313–18.

Larkey, L. K., D. J. Roe, K. L. Weihs, R. Jahnke, A. M. Lopez, C. E. Rogers, B. Oh, and J. Guillen-Rodriguez. "Randomized Controlled Trial of Qigong/Tai Chi Easy on Cancer-Related Fatigue in Breast Cancer Survivors." *Annals of Behavioral Medicine,* August 15, 2014. [Epub ahead of print]

Lasselin, J., S. Lavé, S. Dexpert, A. Aubert, C. Gonzalez, H. Gin, and L. Capuron. "Fatigue Symptoms Relate to Systemic Inflammation in Patients with Type 2 Diabetes." *Brain, Behavior, and Immunity* 26, no. 8 (November 2012): 1211–19.

Lee, Y. C., M. L. Frits, C. K. Iannaccone, M. E. Weinblatt, N. A. Shadick, D. A. Williams, and J. Cui. "Subgrouping of Patients with Rheumatoid Arthritis Based on Pain, Fatigue, Inflammation, and Psychosocial Factors." *Arthritis & Rheumatology* 66, no. 8 (August 2014): 2006–14.

Lindeberg, S. I., M. Rosvall, B. Choi, C. Canivet, S. O. Isacsson, R. Karasek, and P. O. Ostergren. "Psychosocial Working Conditions and Exhaustion in a Working Population Sample of Swedish Middle-Aged Men and Women." *European Journal of Public Health* 21, no. 2 (April 2011): 190–96.

Liptan, G., S. Mist, C. Wright, A. Arzt, and K. D. Jones. "A Pilot Study of Myofascial Release Therapy Compared to Swedish Massage in Fibromyalgia." *Journal of Bodywork and Movement Therapies* 17, no. 3 (July 2013): 365–70.

Loy, B. D., P. J. O'Connor, and R. K. Dishman. "The Effect of a Single Bout of Exercise on Energy and Fatigue States: A Systematic Review and Meta-Analysis." *Fatigue: Biomedicine, Health & Behavior* 1, no. 4 (2013): 223–42.

McEwen, B., and E. Lasley. *The End of Stress As We Know It.* Washington, DC: National Academies Press, 2002.

McInnis, O. A., K. Matheson, and H. Anisman. "Living with the Unexplained: Coping, Distress, and Depression among Women with Chronic Fatigue Syndrome and/or Fibromyalgia Compared to an Autoimmune Disorder." *Anxiety, Stress, and Coping* 27, no. 6 (November 2014): 601–18.

Mengshoel, A. M. "Life Strain-Related Tiredness and Illness-Related Fatigue in Individuals with Ankylosing Spondylitis." *Arthritis Care & Research* 62, no. 9 (September 2010): 1271–77.

Miller, L. R., and A. Cano. "Comorbid Chronic Pain and Depression: Who Is at Risk?" *The Journal of Pain* 10, no. 6 (June 2009): 619–27.

Molassiotis, A., J. Bardy, J. Finnegan-John, P. Mackereth, D. W. Ryder, J. Filshie, E. Ream, and A. Richardson. "Acupuncture for Cancer-Related Fatigue in Patients with Breast Cancer: A Pragmatic Randomized Controlled Trial." *Journal of Clinical Oncology* 30, no. 36 (December 20, 2012): 4470–76.

Morrison, R., and H. Keating III. "Fatigue in Primary Care." *Obstetrics and Gynecology Clinics of North America* 28, no. 2 (2001): 225–40.

National Institute of General Medical Sciences. "Circadian Rhythms Fact Sheet." Content reviewed November 2012.

National Sleep Foundation. "2007 Sleep in America Poll."

Newton, J. L., and D. E. J. Jones. "Making Sense of Fatigue." *Occupational Medicine* 60, no. 5 (2010): 326–29.

Papadakis, M. A., S. J. McPhee, and M. W. Rabow. *Current Medical Diagnosis & Treatment, 2013.* New York: McGraw-Hill Medical, 2013.

Pellino, G., G. Sciaudone, V. Caserta, G. Candilio, G. S. De Fatico, S. Gagliardi, I. Landino, M. Patturelli, G. Riegler, E. L. Di Caprio, S. Canonico, P. Gritti, and F. Selvaggi. "Fatigue in Inflammatory Bowel Diseases: Relationship with Age and Disease Activity." *International Journal of Surgery* 12, Supplement 2 (2014): S60–63.

Price, J. R., E. Mitchell, E. Tidy, and V. Hunot. "Cognitive Behaviour Therapy for Chronic Fatigue Syndrome in Adults." *Cochrane Database of Systematic Reviews*, July 16, 2008, no. 3: CD001027.

Puetz, T. W., S. S. Flowers, and P. J. O'Connor. "A Randomized Controlled Trial of the Effect of Aerobic Exercise Training on Feelings of Energy and Fatigue in Sedentary Young Adults with Persistent Fatigue." *Psychotherapy and Psychosomatics* 77, no. 3 (2008): 167–74.

Ricci, J. A., E. Chee, A. L. Lorandeau, and J. Berger. "Fatigue in the U.S. Workforce: Prevalence and Implications for Lost Productive Work Time." *Journal of Occupational and Environmental Medicine* 49, no. 1 (2007): 1–10.

Rosenthal, T. C., B. A. Majeroni, R. Pretorius, and K. Malik. "Fatigue: An Overview." *American Family Physician* 78, no. 10 (November 15, 2008): 1173–79.

Schoenleber, M., P. I. Chow, and H. Berenbaum. "Self-Conscious Emotions in Worry and Generalized Anxiety Disorder." *British Journal of Clinical Psychology* 53, no. 3 (September 2014): 299–314.

Sharpe, M., and S. Wessely. "Putting the Rest Cure to Rest—Again." *BMJ* 316, no. 7134 (March 14, 1998): 796–800.

Simrén, M., J. Svedlund, I. Posserud, E. S. Bjornsson, and H. Abrahamsson. "Predictors of Subjective Fatigue in Chronic Gastrointestinal Disease." *Alimentary Pharmacology & Therapeutics* 28, no. 5 (September 1, 2008): 638–47.

Singh, R., and P. M. Kluding. "Fatigue and Related Factors in People with Type 2 Diabetes." *The Diabetes Educator* 39, no. 3 (May–June 2013): 320–26.

Skapinakis, P., G. Lewis, and V. Mavreas. "Temporal Relations between Unexplained Fatigue and Depression: Longitudinal Data from an International Study in Primary Care." *Psychosomatic Medicine* 66, no. 3 (May–June 2004): 330–35.

Swain, M. G. "Fatigue in Chronic Disease." *Clinical Science* 99, no. 1 (July 2000): 1–8.

Torres-Harding, S., and L. A. Jason. "What Is Fatigue?" In *Fatigue as a Window to the Brain*. Edited by John DeLuca. Cambridge: MIT Press, 2005.

Wang, C. "Tai Chi Improves Pain and Functional Status in Adults with Rheumatoid Arthritis: Results of a Pilot Single-Blinded Randomized Controlled Trial." *Medicine and Sport Science* 52 (2008): 218–29.

Wang, S. L., C. H. Chang, L. Y. Hu, S. J. Tsai, A. C. Yang, and Z. H. You. "Risk of Developing Depressive Disorders following Rheumatoid Arthritis: A Nationwide Population-Based Study." *PLoS One* 9, no. 9 (September 16, 2014): e107791.

Wang, W. "Parents' Time with Kids More Rewarding Than Paid Work—And More Exhausting." Pew Research Center, *Social & Demographic Trends,* October 8, 2013.

Watanabe, Y., and K. Hirohiko. "Brain Science on Chronic Fatigue." *Japan Medical Association Journal* 49, no. 1 (January 2006): 19–26.

Yoshihara, K., T. Hiramoto, T. Oka, C. Kubo, and N. Sudo. "Effect of 12 Weeks of Yoga Training on the Somatization, Psychological Symptoms, and Stress-Related Biomarkers of Healthy Women." *BioPsychoSocial Medicine* 8, no. 1 (January 3, 2014): 1.

Zakerimoghadam, M., K. Tavasoli, A. K. Nejad, and S. Khoshkesht. "The Effect of Breathing Exercises on the Fatigue Levels of Patients with Chronic Obstructive Pulmonary Disease." *Acta Medica Indonesiana* 43, no. 1 (January 2011): 29–33.

Index

C

Caffeine
  minimizing intake of, 202
  pros and cons of, <u>67–68</u>
  sleep disturbances from, 31
  as stimulant, xii, <u>67</u>, 227
Calcium supplements, as sleep aid, 36–37, 201
Calming activity, for stress relief, 54
Calories, amount needed, <u>69</u>
Cancer
  breast, <u>82</u>, <u>99</u>
  Epstein-Barr virus linked to, 158
  lung, 125
  mind-body exercise and, <u>82</u>
  reducing fatigue from, 54
  uterine, <u>99</u>
Capsaicin, as stimulant, 228
Carbohydrates, 62, 63, 205
  for breakfast, 66
  snacks with, 72
Cardiac arrhythmias, 122
Cardiac infections, 123–24
Cardiomyopathy, 123
Cardiovascular disease. *See* Heart disease
Carnitine, for energy boost, 229
CBT. *See* Cognitive behavioral therapy
Celiac disease, xii, 137, 142–43
Central sleep apnea, 39
CFS. *See* Chronic fatigue syndrome
Chamomile tea, as sleep aid, 37
Chest stretch, 208
Cholesterol-lowering medications, fatigue from, 224
Chronic disease
  from Epstein-Barr virus, 158
  sleep loss link to, xviii
Chronic fatigue syndrome (CFS), 184
  author's experience with, xiii, xiv, 89, 184
  conditions coexisting with, 144, 154–55, <u>157</u>
  depression and, xiv, <u>182</u>
  diagnosing, 18, 152–53, 156
  Epstein-Barr virus linked to, 158, 159
  exercise and, 81, 89

improvement of, 156
  incidence of, 152
  increased acceptance of, 13
  migraines and, 172
  probiotics for, <u>140</u>
  squelched feelings and, <u>189</u>
  symptoms of, 12, 15, 151, 152–53, 155, 156, <u>160</u>, 165, 184
  treating, 155, 156
    caution about, 156, 158
  triggers of, 152, 153–54
  varying severity of, 155
Chronic kidney disease (CKD)
  causes of, 134
  conditions coexisting with, 121
  diagnosing, 134–35
  incidence of, 132
  symptoms of, 132–34
  treating, 134, 135
Chronic obstructive pulmonary disease (COPD), 125–26, 207
Circadian rhythms, 17, 30
Cirrhosis, 127, 128
  primary biliary, 128–29
CKD. *See* Chronic kidney disease
Clean-eating plan, 201–5
Coenzyme Q10, for energy boost, 228
Cognitive behavioral therapy (CBT), for treating
  anxiety disorders, 25, <u>55</u>, 194
  chronic fatigue syndrome, 155, 156
  depression, 185, 186
  insomnia, 36
  irritable bowel syndrome, 145
  stress, <u>55–56</u>, 57
  unexplained fatigue, 20
Cognitive dietary restraint, 59–60
Cognitive flip, for stress relief, 56–57
Colorful foods, antioxidants in, 70
Colors, energizing, <u>215–16</u>
Complex sleep apnea, 39
Compulsive exercise disorder, 86–87
Congenital heart defects, 122
Constipation
  with irritable bowel syndrome, 144
  probiotics for, <u>140</u>
COPD, 125–26, 207

Dopamine
    antidepressants altering, 186
    in fibromyalgia sufferers, 168
    in gut vs. brain, 138
Dysthymia, 179, 183

E

Eating disorders, 64–65
Eating habits. *See also* Diet; Food
    clean, 201–5
    effect on energy, 60–61
    poor, 59–60
    stress and, 48
EBV. *See* Epstein-Barr virus
Edlund, Matthew, 33
EGCG, in green tea, 228
Electroconvulsive therapy, for treatment-
        resistant depression, 191
Electrolyte disturbances, with chronic
        kidney disease, 133
Electronic devices
    sleep disturbances from, 32, 49
    stress from, 49
Emotional habits, bad, breaking, 188–90
Emphysema, 126–27
Endocarditis, 124
Endocrine disorders
    adrenal disorders, 102–4
    fatigue from, 96
    polycystic ovary syndrome, 95–96
    thyroid disorders, xii, 100–102, 193
    type 2 diabetes, 97–100 (*see also*
        Diabetes)
Endocrine symptoms checklist, 214
Endocrine system, functions of, 93–94
Endorphins, exercise boosting, 52, 78
Energy
    adenosine triphosphate and, 61–62
    analogy about, 16
    from caffeine (*see* Caffeine)
    eating habits increasing, 66, 68, 70, 72–76
    eating habits reducing, 60–61, 64–65,
        67, 73
    exercise for, 10, 77–78, 79, 80–83
    food providing, 59, 62–64, 74–76
        (*see also* Diet)

hormones influencing, 93, 94
lifestyle depleting, 17–18
quick boosters of, 215–16
regaining, after treating fatigue, xv
sleep conserving, 27
supplements boosting, 227–29
Epsom salt bath, as sleep aid, 201
Epstein-Barr virus (EBV), 19, 158–61
    diseases linked to, 108, 153
Essential fatty acids, 160. *See also*
        Omega-3 fatty acids
Estrogen
    fluctuations in, 17, 28, 93
    infection boosted by, 107
Estrogen dominance, from overweight,
        99
Exercise(s). *See also* Physical activity;
        Walking
    best time for, 32, 53
    energy from, 10, 77–78, 79, 80–83
    excessive, effects of, 86–89
    guidelines for, 83–85
    health benefits of, 78–80
    mind-body, 82
    proper breathing for, 84
    for relieving
        depression, 186
        fibromyalgia pain, 171
        postviral fatigue, 160
        stress, 52, 53, 57
        unexplained fatigue, 20
    starting, 89
    strength training, 81, 85
    stretching, 207–8
Exercise buddy, 85
Exhaustion. *See* Fatigue
Exhaustion epidemic, xii, xiii

F

Fasting blood sugar test, 98
Fasts, juice, 70–71
Fatigue
    analyzing symptoms of, 210–14
    author's experience with, xi–xii,
        xiii–xiv, xviii–xix, 55, 89, 184,
        219

Gastrointestinal symptoms checklist, 212
Gastrointestinal tract
  bacteria in, 138–39
  as second brain, 138
Generalized anxiety disorder (GAD), 188, 192, 194
Genitourinary symptoms checklist, 212
GERD. *See* Gastroesophageal reflux disease
Gluten intolerance
  in celiac disease, 142–43
  fatigue from, 18
Goji berries, for energy boost, 75
Graves' disease, 102, 106
Green drinks, 202–3
Green tea, as stimulant, 228
Guillain-Barré syndrome, infections linked to, 108
Guilt trips, overcoming, 188–89

H

Hamstring stretch, 208
Harris-Benedict equation, 69
Hashimoto's thyroiditis, 101, 103
Headaches, migraine, 171–74
Head symptoms checklist, 211
Heart and circulation symptoms checklist, 212
Heartburn, chronic. *See* Gastroesophageal reflux disease
Heart defects, congenital, 122
Heart disease
  causes of, xviii, 121–22
  deaths from, 121
  incidence of, 121
  symptoms of, 119, 121, 122
Heart failure, 122
Heart medications, fatigue-causing, 124
Heart problems
  symptoms of, 119, 120
  types of, 121–24
Heavy meals, avoiding, before bedtime, 30
Hemochromatosis, 130
Hemoglobin A1C test, 98
Hepatitis, 131–32
Herbal sleep remedies, 37
Herpes virus, 153, 158, 159, 161

High blood pressure, chronic kidney disease from, 134
Histamine (H2) blockers
  fatigue from, 141, 145
  for GERD, 145, 146
Hormonal imbalances. *See also* Endocrine disorders
  with chronic fatigue syndrome, 153
  symptoms of, 94
  treating, 104
Hormonal shifts
  fatigue from, 17
  during menstrual cycle, 17, 27–28, 93
  sleep disruptions from, 27–28
Hormones. *See also specific hormones*
  appetite-regulating, 27
  endocrine system producing, 93–94
  released during sleep, 26
  reproductive, effects on energy, 93
HPA axis, 14, 46, 48
H2 blockers, 141, 145, 146
Hydration, water for, 72–73, 208–9
Hyperthyroidism, 101–2, 122
Hyponatremia, 209
Hypothalamic-pituitary-adrenal (HPA) axis, 14, 46, 48
Hypothyroidism, 15, 100–101

I

IBD. *See* Inflammatory bowel disease
IBS. *See* Irritable bowel syndrome
Immune system
  autoimmune diseases and, 106, 117
    (*see also* Autoimmune diseases)
  functions of, 105
  infections and, 149, 150
Immunity, natural vs. acquired, 105
Immunotherapy, for autoimmune diseases, 113
Infections
  as autoimmune disease trigger, 107, 108
  cardiac, 123–24
  chronic fatigue syndrome, 151–56, 158
  diagnosing, 164
  Epstein-Barr virus, 108, 153, 158–61

treating, 111
virus linked to, 108
Lyme disease, 162–64
Lyrica (pregabalin), for fibromyalgia, 170, 171

M

Macronutrients, 62, 66. *See also* Carbohydrates; Fats, dietary; Protein
Magnesium, sources of, 203
Magnesium deficiency, 76, 203
Magnesium supplements, as sleep aid, 36–37, 201
Major depressive disorder (MDD), 180, 182–83, 184, 185, 187. *See also* Depression
Mantra, for exercise, 85
Massage therapy, xviii, 20, 171, 175, 187
McEwen, Bruce, 47
MCS (multiple chemical sensitivity), 154, 157
MDD. *See* Major depressive disorder
Meal frequency, 204–5
Meals, heavy, bedtime and, 30
Meal timing, 68
Medical conditions
as cause of fatigue, 12, 18, 19 (*see also specific diseases and conditions*)
insomnia from, 35
Medications. *See also specific medications*
effect on gut bacteria, 139
fatigue-causing, 18, 19, 124, 141, 145, 223–25
insomnia from, 35
for migraine prevention, 173–74
restless legs syndrome from, 41
for treating
anxiety disorders, 194
arthritis, 174, 175
depression (*see* Antidepressants)
diabetes, 99
fibromyalgia, 170, 171
GERD, 141, 145, 146
inflammatory bowel disease, 147

insomnia, 36, 37–38
irritable bowel syndrome, 144–45
lupus, 111
migraines, 173
restless legs syndrome, 42
rheumatoid arthritis, 112
sinus infections, 162
treatment-resistant depression, 187, 191
Meditation
for depression treatment, 187
for stress relief, 54
Mediterranean diet, 66
Melatonin, light suppressing, 49, 201, 216
Melatonin supplements, as sleep aid, 36
Men
less fatigue in, xii
sleep apnea in, 39
Menopause
hormones and, 28, 93, 99
sleep disturbances in, 28
Menstrual cycle, hormonal shifts during, 17, 27–28, 93
Mental-health symptoms checklist, 213
Mental rest, 33
Metabolic syndrome, 99–100, 128
Micronutrients, 63, 66
Migraines, 171–74
Mind-body exercises, 82
Minerals, in foods, 63
Mini-meals, 204–5
Mitochondria, exercise producing, 78
Mixed sleep apnea, 39
Modafinil, for unexplained fatigue, 20
Mononucleosis, xiii, 158
Mothers, fatigue of, xii
Motivation, for exercise, 85
Mouth guard, for treating
sleep apnea, 40, 41
temporomandibular joint disorder, 177
Multiple chemical sensitivity (MCS), 154, 157
Multiple sclerosis, 108, 115–16, 143, 175

Muscle pain, fatigue with, 165–66
Muscle relaxants, for insomnia, 38
Musculoskeletal symptoms checklist, 213
Music, for energy boost, <u>216</u>
Myasthenia gravis, viruses linked to, 108
Myocarditis, 108, 123–24
Myofascial release, for fibromyalgia pain, 171

N

Naps, 32, 34
NASH (nonalcoholic steatohepatitis), 127–28
Natural Calm, as sleep aid, 36–37, 201
Natural immunity, 105
Natural light
    for energy boost, <u>215</u>
    for sleep improvement, 30
Neck pain, 165, 177–78
Neck stretch, 207
Negative thinking, stress from, <u>56</u>
Nephrons, kidney, 132
Neurofeedback training, for stress relief, 55
Neurologic symptoms checklist, 213
Neurotransmitters
    factors altering
        antidepressants, 185
        caffeine, <u>67</u>
        depression, 175
        exercise, 52, 78
        fibromyalgia, 14, 168
        pain, 166
        sleep disorders, 169
    in gut vs. brain, 138
    sleep-inducing, 37
Niacin, for energy boost, 229
Nicotine, sleep disturbances from, 31
Nonalcoholic fatty liver disease, 121, 127–28
Nonalcoholic steatohepatitis (NASH), 127–28
Nonsteroidal anti-inflammatory drugs. *See* NSAIDs

Norepinephrine
    antidepressants and, 186
    chronic pain and, 166
    in fibromyalgia sufferers, 168
NSAIDs
    GERD and, 146
    kidney damage from, 134, 173
    for treating
        arthritis, 175
        lupus, 111
        migraines, 173
        rheumatoid arthritis, 112
        Sjögren's syndrome, 114
        temporomandibular joint disorders, 177
Nutrient absorption, disorders reducing, 139–41
Nutrient deficiencies, 63, 203–4

O

Oats, for energy boost, 74
Obesity. *See* Overweight and obesity
Obstructive sleep apnea, 39
Omega-3 fatty acids
    for arthritis, 175
    for depression relief, 187
    food sources of, 71, 75, 204
    health benefits of, 62, 71, 204
ORAC value, 70
Organ dysfunctions
    chronic kidney disease, 121, 132–35
    fatigue with, 120–21, 135
    heart problems, 119, 120, 121–24
    liver diseases, 120, 121, 127–32
    lung diseases, 120, 125–27
Organs, routine functioning of, 120
Orthorexia, <u>65</u>
Osteoarthritis, 174
OTS (overtraining syndrome), 86
Overexercising, 86–89
Overtraining syndrome (OTS), 86
Overweight and obesity
    estrogen overload from, <u>99</u>
    low energy with, 60
    sleep apnea and, 39

P

Pain, chronic
  depression from, 166
  fatigue with, 165–66
  managing, 178
Painful conditions
  arthritis, 174–76
  back, neck, and shoulder pain, 177–78
  fibromyalgia (*see* Fibromyalgia)
  migraines, 171–74
  temporomandibular joint disorders,
    176–77
Pain medications, for insomnia, 38
PBC (primary biliary cirrhosis), 128–29
PCOS (polycystic ovary syndrome),
    95–96
People pleasing, overcoming, 189–90
Perfectionism, overcoming, 188
Pericarditis, 123
Perimenopause, hormonal shifts during,
    17
Periodic limb movement disorder
    (PLMD), 41, 42
Pernicious anemia, 116–17
Personalized energy-boosting plan, xviii,
    10, 199–214. *See also* 7-day
    fatigue-beating challenge
Pets, sleep disturbances from, 34
Physical activity. *See also* Exercise(s)
  inadequate, 20
  preventing depression, 179–80
Physical rest, 33
Plaquenil, for treating
  lupus, 110, 111
  rheumatoid arthritis, 112
  Sjögren's syndrome, 114
PLMD (periodic limb movement
    disorder), 41, 42
PMS, 17, 28
Polycystic ovary syndrome (PCOS),
    95–96
Polysomnography, 40
Positive thinking, for stress relief, 57
Post-traumatic stress disorder (PTSD)
  exercise relieving, 52
  as fibromyalgia trigger, 168

Post-treatment Lyme disease syndrome
    (PTLDS), 163, 164
Posture, 215
Postviral fatigue, 160
PPIs. *See* Proton pump inhibitors
Pregabalin, for fibromyalgia, 170, 171
Pregnancy
  autoimmune diseases after, 107–8
  sleep disturbances during, 28
Primary biliary cirrhosis (PBC), 128–29
Probiotics, 140, 144, 205
Progesterone, 17, 28, 93
Protein, 62, 63, 205
  for breakfast, 66
  in snacks, 72
  sources of, 74, 75, 76
Proton pump inhibitors (PPIs)
  fatigue from, 141, 145, 225
  for GERD, 145, 146
Psychotherapy
  for anxiety disorder, 194
  for depression, 184, 185, 186, 187
PTLDS (post-treatment Lyme disease
    syndrome), 163, 164
PTSD (post-traumatic stress disorder)
  exercise relieving, 52
  as fibromyalgia trigger, 168

Q

Qigong, 82
Quad and hip flexor stretch, 208
Questionnaires, about cause of fatigue,
    4–9, 19
  interpreting, 9–10
Quinoa, for energy boost, 74

R

RA. *See* Rheumatoid arthritis
Relaxation techniques, for stress relief, 54
REM sleep, 26, 43, 73
Respiratory infections, 126, 161
Respiratory symptoms checklist, 212
Rest, types of, 33

Restless legs syndrome (RLS), 35, 41–42
Rheumatoid arthritis (RA)
  depression with, 174–75
  diagnosing, 112
  incidence of, 111
  infections linked to, 108
  positive thinking and, 57
  symptoms of, xii, 106, 107, 111, 165, 174
  tai chi for, 82
  treating, 112–13, 175, 176
RLS (restless legs syndrome), 35, 41–42
Rumination, overcoming, 190
Runners' high, 78

S

Salmon, for energy boost, 75
Saying no, for stress relief, 53–54
Second shift, of women, 48, 50
Sedentary lifestyle, 77, 78, 79–80
Serotonin
  factors altering
    antidepressants, 186
    chronic pain, 166
    exercise, 78
    fatigue from, 13
    fibromyalgia, 168
    hormonal shifts, 17
    sleep disorders, 169
  in gut vs. brain, 138
  for sleep improvement, 37, 201
7-day fatigue-beating challenge, xviii, 10, 199
  strategies in
    body-tension inventory, 206–8
    clean-foods diet, 201–5
    fatigue diary, 200
    sleeping alone, 200–201
    symptoms analysis, 210–14
    "to-don't" list, 209–10
    walking for 10 minutes, 205–6
    water drinking, 208–9
Shoulder pain, 177–78
Shoulder stretch, 207
Sinus infections, 153, 161–62
Sitting, health effects of, 77, 78, 79–80

Sjögren's syndrome, 113–15, 143
Skin symptoms checklist, 213
SLE. *See* Lupus
Sleep
  determining needed amount of, 29–30
  hormonal shifts and, 27–28
  improving (*see* Sleep hygiene)
  restorative effects of, 26–27, 42
  rest vs., 33
  stages of, 42–43
Sleep aids
  natural, 36–37, 201
  over-the-counter, 36
  prescription, 37–38
Sleep apnea, 35, 39–41
  author's experience with, xiii, xiv, 34, 41
Sleep deprivation
  from anxiety, 191
  with depression, 180
  effects of, xviii, 25, 26, 29
    energy depletion, 17–18
  health risks from, 27
  in modern culture, 25–26
  in women, xii, 27–29, 35–36
Sleep disorders
  fibromyalgia-related, 169
  incidence of, 34–35
  insomnia, 28, 35–38
  restless legs syndrome, 35, 41–42
  seeking help for, 34, 36, 40, 42
  sleep apnea, 34, 35, 39–41
  snoring and, 38–39, 40
  types of, 35
Sleep hygiene, 10, 29–32, 34, 200–201
Sleep schedule, importance of, 30
Smoking, sleep disturbances from, 31
Snacks
  benefits of, 71–72
  good choices of, 72
  sleep-inducing, 30–31
Snoring, 38–39, 40
Social rest, 33
Spiritual rest, 33
Statin drugs, fatigue from, 124, 224
Stimulating activities, sleep disturbances from, 32
Strength training, 81, 85

Stress
    chronic, 45
        effects of, 46–48
    chronic fatigue syndrome and, 153, 154
    cortisol increased by, 46, 47, 60, 94
    energy depletion from, 18, 82
    fatigue from, xii, 46, 48, 50–51
    as fibromyalgia trigger, 168
    gut bacteria and, 138
    IBS flares from, 145
    managing, 10, 51–58
    physiological effects of, 46
    sleep problems and, 27, 28–29
    sources of, 45, 49
    types of, 45
    of women, 47, 48, 50
Stress hormones. *See also* Adrenaline;
        Cortisol
    effect on brain structure, 193
    factors releasing
        anxiety, 191
        chronic stress, 46, 47
        overtraining syndrome, 86
Stress response, 46, 48, 55, 107, 141
Stretching exercises, 207–8
Stroke, linked to sleep loss, xviii
Substance P, in fibromyalgia sufferers, 14
Superfoods, energy-boosting, 74–76
Superwoman myth, xvi, 9, 188
Supplements
    adrenal fatigue, caution about, 103
    ASU, for arthritis, 175
    caution with, 20, 229
    energy-boosting, 227–29
    iron, 204
    probiotic, 140, 144, 205
    sleep-aid, 36–37, 201
Symptom inventory, 104, 210–14
Syndrome X. *See* Metabolic syndrome
Systemic lupus erythematosis (SLE).
        See Lupus

T

Tai chi, 54, 81, 82, 126
Tea(s)
    green, as stimulant, 228
    herbal, as sleep aid, 37

Technology
    sleep disturbances from, 32, 49
    stress from, 49
Telomere shortening, 48
Temporomandibular joint disorders
        (TMD), 176–77
Testosterone, infection suppressed by, 107
Testosterone imbalances
    in PCOS, 95
    symptoms of, 93
Thayer, Robert, 205
Thiamin, for energy boost, 229
Thyroid disorders, xii, 100–102, 193
Thyroiditis, 102, 106
Tick bites, Lyme disease from, 162–64
Time management, for stress relief, 53–54
Tiredness, vs. fatigue, 12
TMD (temporomandibular joint
        disorder), 176–77
"To-don't" lists, 53–54, 209–10
Transcranial magnetic stimulation, for
        treatment-resistant depression, 191
Triglycerides, elevated, 128
Tryptophan, fatigue and, 13
Turkey, for energy boost, 75

U

Ulcerative colitis, 141, 142, 147–48
Unexplained fatigue, 12, 18, 19–20
Upper-back stretch, 207
Urinary tract infections (UTIs), 150, 151
Uterine cancer, 99

V

Vagus nerve stimulation, for treatment-
        resistant depression, 191
Valacyclovir, for Epstein-Barr virus, 159,
        161
Valerian tea, as sleep aid, 37
Vegetable-juice fasts, 70–71
Vegetables, antioxidants in, 70
Viruses
    Epstein-Barr, 19, 108, 153, 158–61
    herpes, 153, 158, 159, 161
    prolonged fatigue after, 160